Therapy Approaches in Neurological Disorders

Edited by Mario Bernardo-Filho, Redha Taiar, Danúbia da Cunha de Sá-Caputo and Adérito Seixas

Published in London, United Kingdom

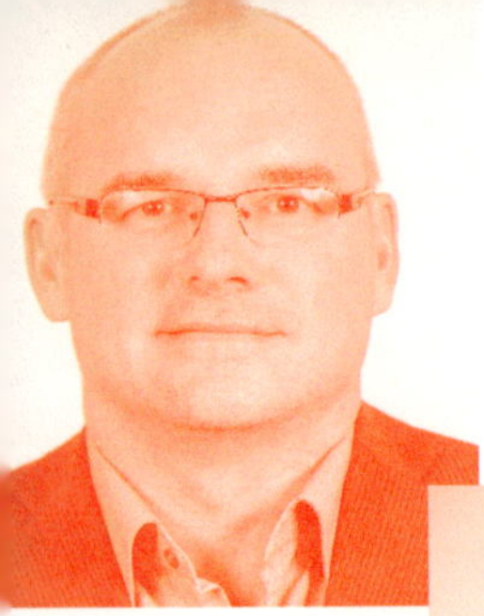
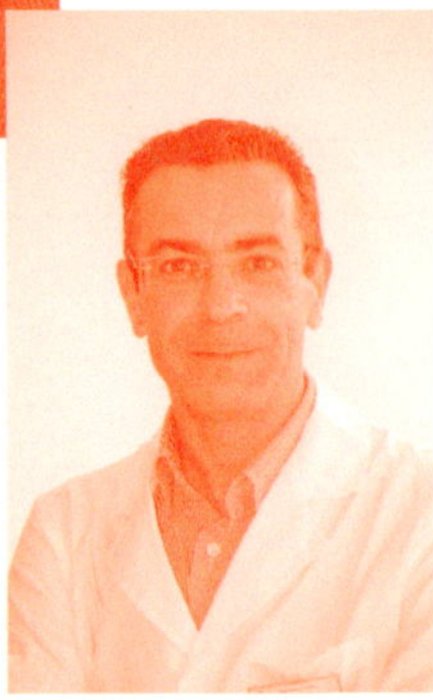
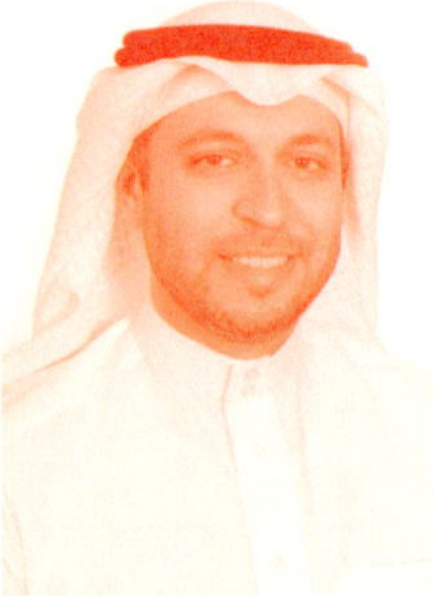
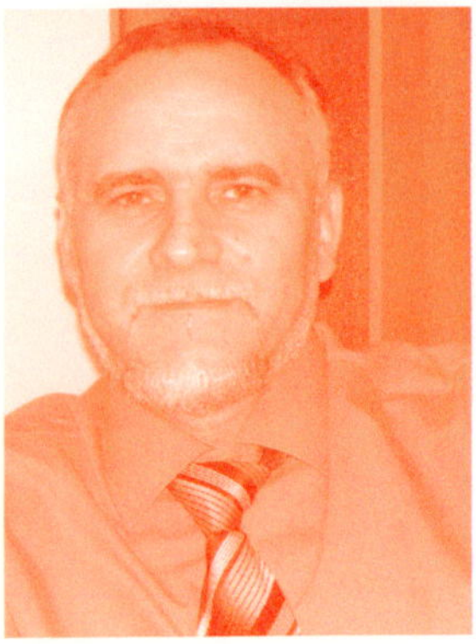
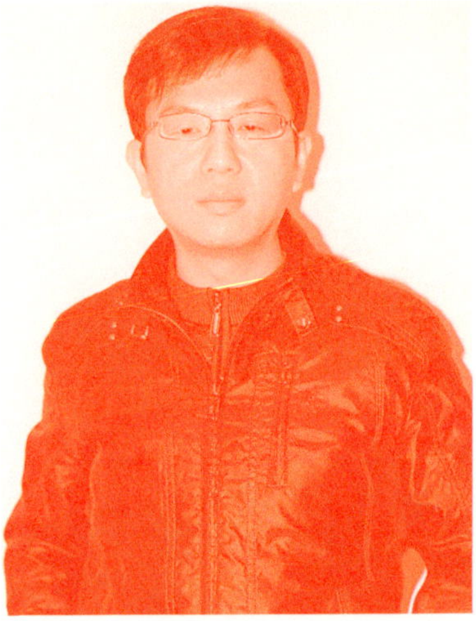
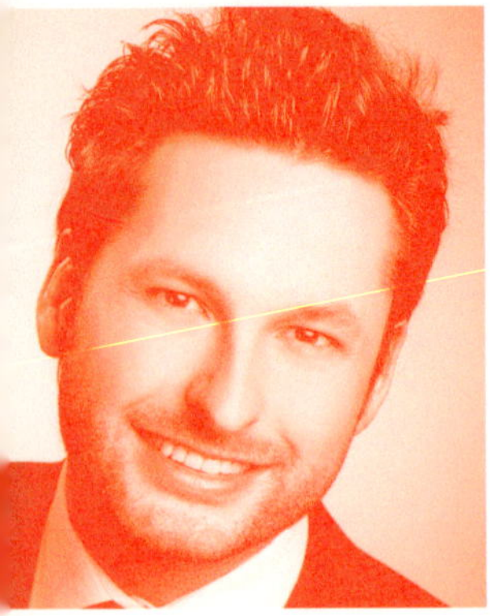
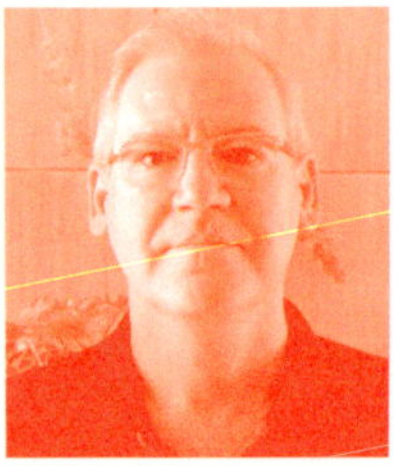

IntechOpen

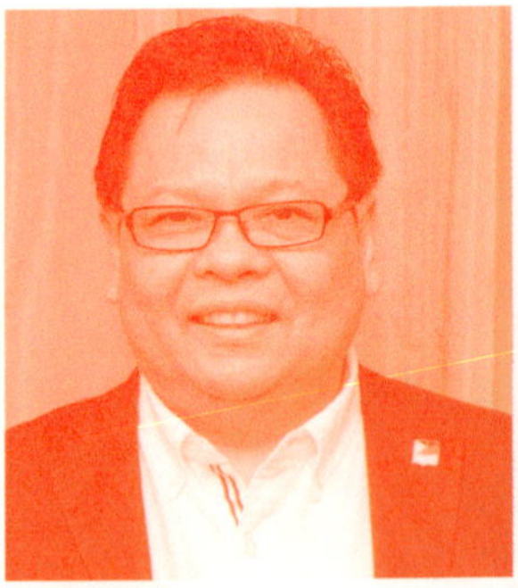
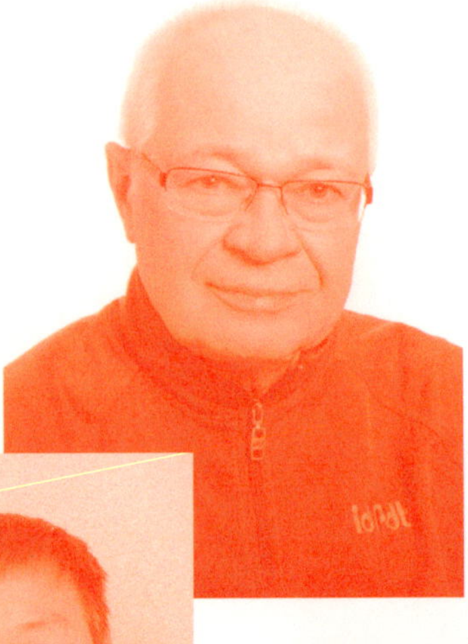
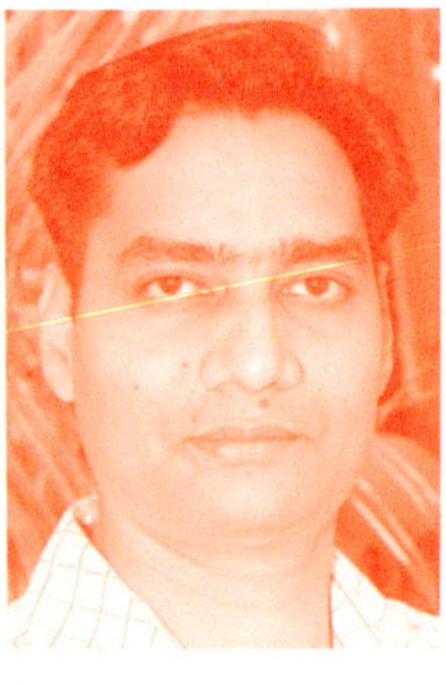
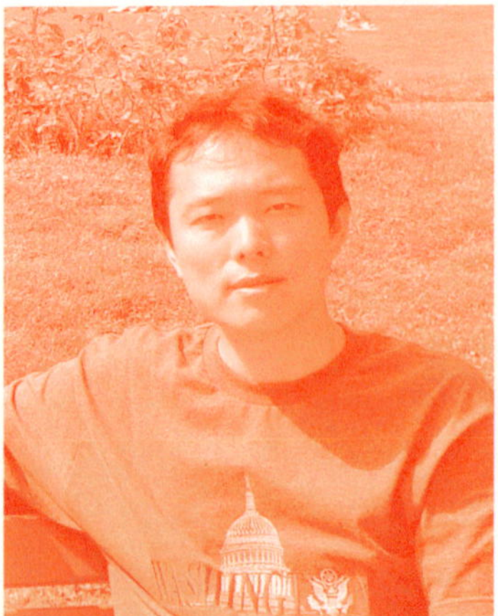
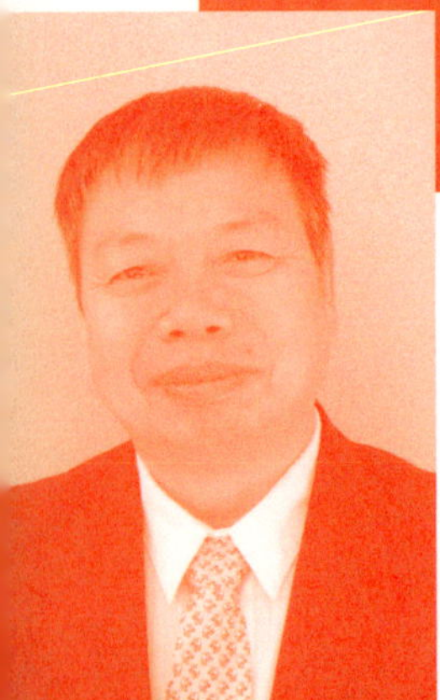
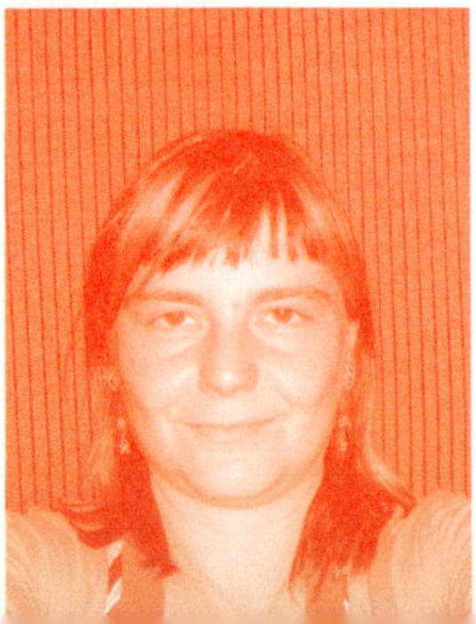

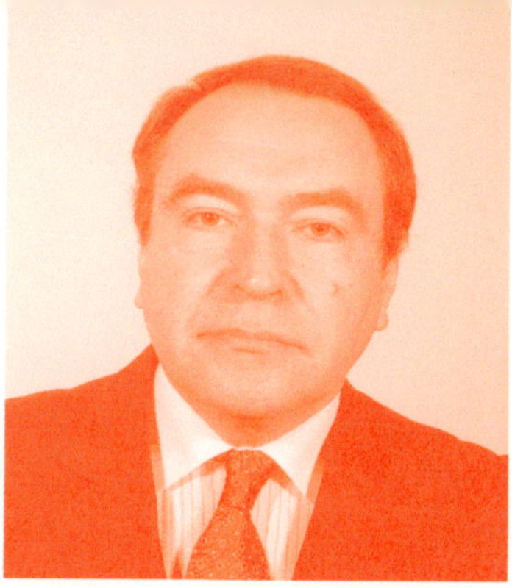
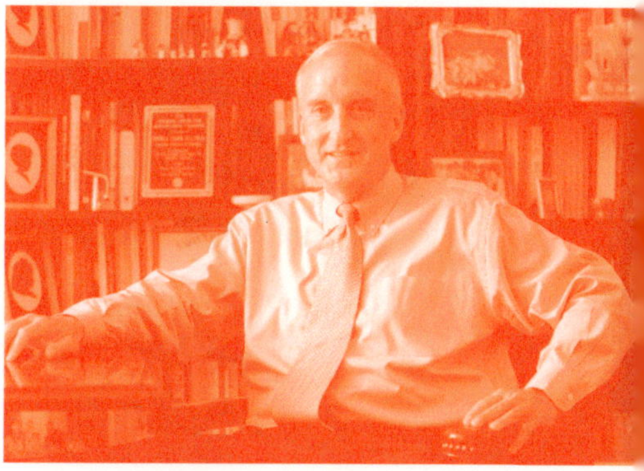
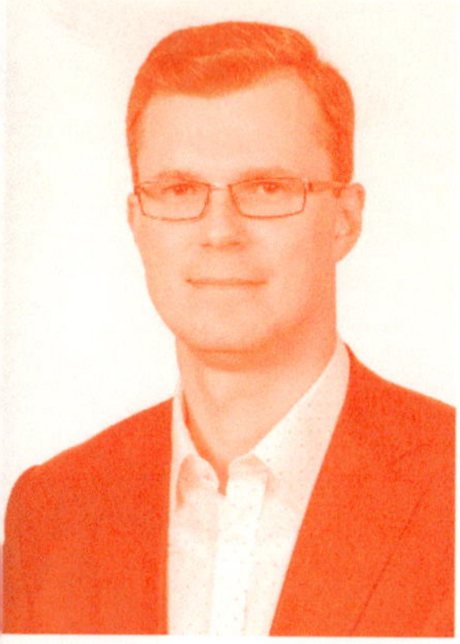
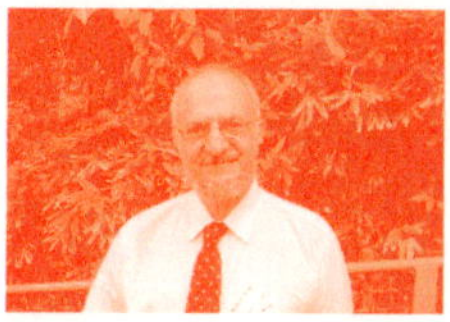
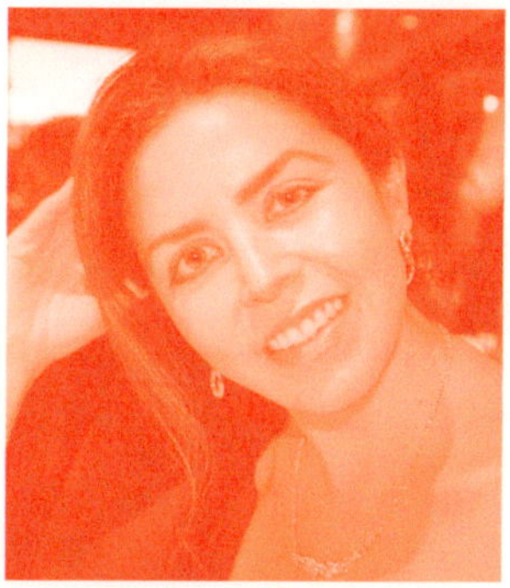

Supporting open minds since 2005

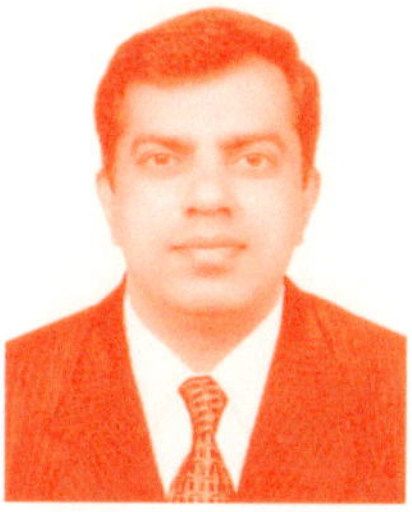
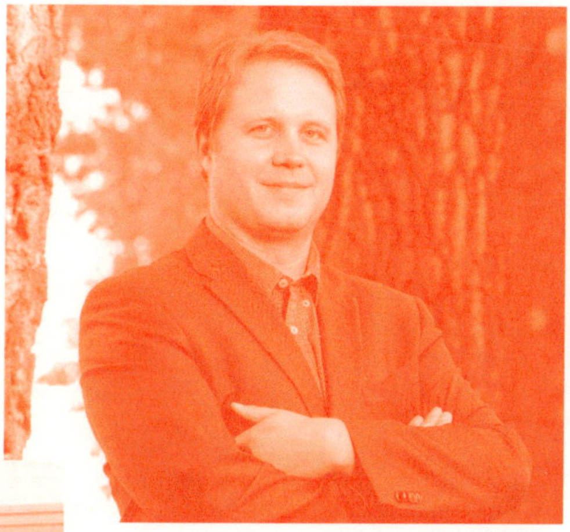
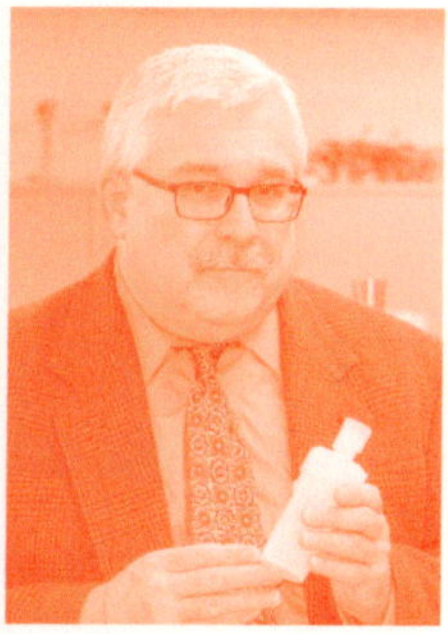
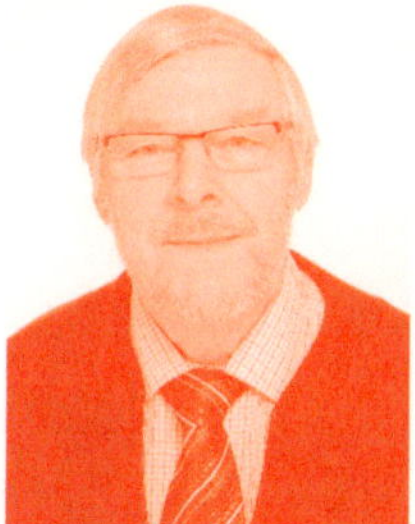
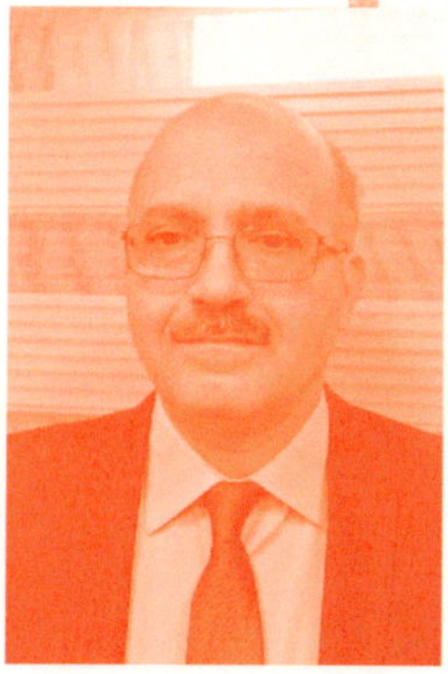
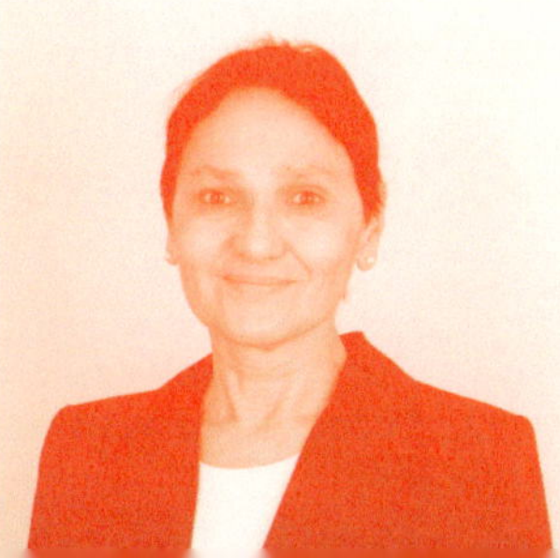
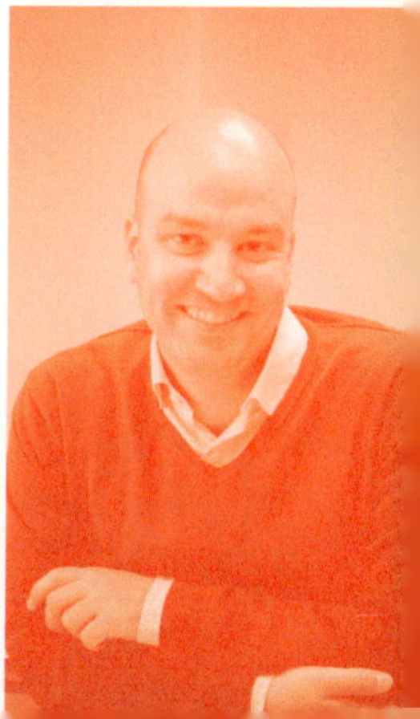

Therapy Approaches in Neurological Disorders
http://dx.doi.org/10.5772/intechopen.91533
Edited by Mario Bernardo-Filho, Redha Taiar, Danúbia da Cunha de Sá-Caputo and Adérito Seixas

Contributors
Vadim I. Ershov, Terry Ellapen, Adele Jordaan, Mariette Swanepoel, Yvonne Paul, Katherine Quiñones, Aydee Robayo, Paul A. Oakley, Ibrahim M. Moustafa, Deed E. Harrison, Noureddine Chaachouay, Lahcen Zidane, James P. Patrick Dickey, Liliana Alvarez, James W.G. Thompson, Marquise M. Bonn, Tahani K. K. Alshammari, Nouf M. Alrasheed, Lina Alhushan, Reema Alhoutah, Anfal F. Bin Dayel, Asma S. Alonazi, Musaad A. Alshammari, Mario Bernardo-Filho, Redha Taiar, Adérito Seixas, Danúbia Da Cunha De Sá-Caputo

First published in London, United Kingdom, 2021 by IntechOpen
IntechOpen is the global imprint of INTECHOPEN LIMITED, registered in England and Wales, registration number: 11086078, 5 Princes Gate Court, London, SW7 2QJ, United Kingdom
Printed in Croatia

British Library Cataloguing-in-Publication Data
A catalogue record for this book is available from the British Library

Additional hard and PDF copies can be obtained from orders@intechopen.com

Therapy Approaches in Neurological Disorders
Edited by Mario Bernardo-Filho, Redha Taiar, Danúbia da Cunha de Sá-Caputo and Adérito Seixas
p. cm.
Print ISBN 978-1-83968-668-9
Online ISBN 978-1-83968-669-6
eBook (PDF) ISBN 978-1-83968-670-2

For EU product safety concerns:
IN TECH d.o.o., Prolaz Marije Krucifikse Kozulić 3, 51000 Rijeka, Croatia, info@intechopen.com or visit our website at intechopen.com.

Meet the editors

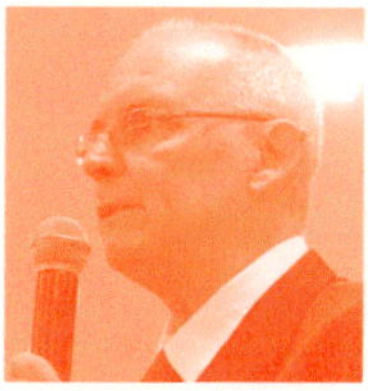

Mario Bernardo-Filho is the head of the Laboratório de Vibrações Mecânicas e Práticas Integrativas-LAVIMPI, Instituto de Biologia Roberto Alcantara Gomes, Departamento de Biofísica e Biometria, and Policlínica Piquet Carneiro, Universidade do Estado do Rio de Janeiro (UERJ). He completed academic courses in Biomedicine and Physiotherapy and obtained his Ph.D. in 1988. In 1999, he participated in a competition to become a full professor at UERJ. He supervises research since 2010 involving integrative and complementary medicine (auriculotherapy and acupuncture) and mechanical vibrations generated in vibrating platforms that produce whole-body vibration exercises (WBVE) when a subject is in contact with a vibrating platform. Studies to evaluate the consequences of WBVE and extracts of medicinal plants in rats are ongoing, as are investigations about the effects of WBVE in individuals with different diseases as well as healthy people. Dr. Bernardo-Filho supervises masters of science and Ph.D. theses. He has participated in and lectured at various national and international congresses. He is editor in chief of the *Brazilian Journal of Health and Biomedical Sciences*, and guest editor of some scientific journals. He is also a reviewer for several scientific journals indexed in PubMed and Scopus.

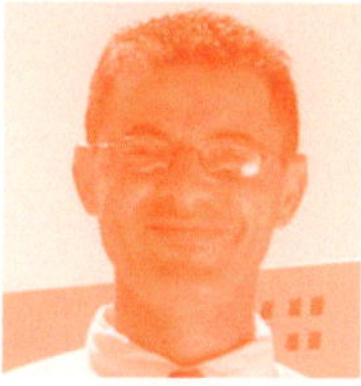

Prof. Redha Taiar has a Ph.D. in Biomechanics and is a professor at the University of Reims Champagne-Ardenne (URCA). He has been head of the European Master of Biomechanics, Ergonomics and Clinical Research; the university diplomas of Podiatrics and Ergonomics; the Laboratory of Biomechanics at the University of Reims; and the Redha Taiar Biomechanical Engineering Society (RTBE) developed for sport and medical advice for the industry. He has been also the vice head of the Department of Sport Science (University of Reims). His research focuses on industry engineering for medicine and high-level sports. He is a specialist in biomechanics, health disease, and rehabilitation. His researches publications can be found at:
https://publons.com/researcher/Q-6769-2016/
https://orcid.org/0000-0002-0227-3884
https://pubmed.ncbi.nlm.nih.gov/?term=taiar+r
https://www.scopus.com/authid/detail.uri?authorId=15823162100
https://www.researchgate.net/profile/Redha_Taiar
https://scholar.google.fr/citations?user=2FP-NPQAAAAJ&hl=fr&oi=ao

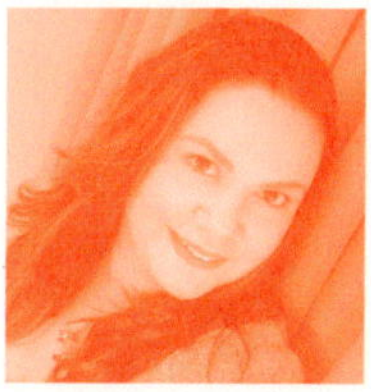

Dr. Danúbia da Cunha de Sá-Caputo graduated in Physiotherapy with a specialization in Acupuncture. She received an MSc from Rio de Janeiro State University, Brazil, for a thesis focused on the use of whole-body vibration exercise in cerebral palsy and metabolic syndrome patients. She received a Ph.D. from the same university for a thesis focused on the use of whole-body vibration exercises in chronic diseases. She is pursuing her post-doctorate at the Laboratório de Vibrações Mecânicas e Práticas Integrativas, Rio de Janeiro State University. She is a professor and the head of a scientific research group at the Bezerra de Araújo Faculty, Brazil. She is a vice-president of Associação Brasileira de

Fisioterapia Integrativa e Práticas Integrativas e Complementares em Saúde, Brazil. She is also a supervisor of graduate, MSc, and Ph.D. students. She is a reviewer and editorial board member of scientific journals.

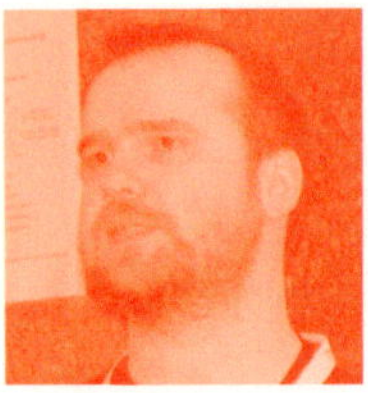

Dr. Adérito Seixas graduated in Physiotherapy with a specialization in Neuromusculoskeletal Rehabilitation. He received his MSc from the University of Porto, Portugal, for a thesis on the assessment of sensorimotor skills of athletes with and without disabilities. He also specialized in data analysis at the same university. He is the president of the Portuguese Association of Physiotherapists, a board member of the European Association of Thermology, and a member of several scientific societies. Currently, alongside his work as a full-time professor of a graduate course on Physiotherapy and a master's program at Escola Superior de Saúde, Universidade Fernando Pessoa, Porto, Portugal, he is carrying out research for his Ph.D., focusing on the biomechanical and thermophysiological assessment of the foot in diabetic patients at risk of developing foot ulcers. His research interests lie in evidence-based practice, assessment of the neuromusculoskeletal system, and the role of cognitive assessment in human adaptation to performance situations.

Contents

Preface

Neurological disorders and related sequelae affect an important number of individuals worldwide with generally catastrophic consequences to quality of life and wellbeing. Individuals with neurological conditions often experience negative consequences such as social and economic burdens, often implying social exclusion and discrimination. This book contributes to the understanding and management of some neurological disorders. It is divided into four sections exploring nonpharmacological and pharmacological interventions and other approaches to managing neurological conditions.

The first section includes an introductory chapter that covers various topics with high relevance in the field of neurological disorders.

The second section includes chapters on the relevance and impact of whole-body vibration exercise, biofeedback, and sagittal plane spine alignment on people with neurological conditions. Whole-body vibration exercise is a safe management tool and biofeedback has proven to reduce the severity of post-concussive symptoms. Sagittal spine alignment restoration plays a relevant role in improving neurophysiology, sensorimotor control, and autonomic nervous system function.

The third section includes a chapter on how a prototype for a standing device in children with spinal dysraphism seems to facilitate the maintenance of a standing position. It also includes chapters on the complications of dysphagia in individuals with neurological disorders and the relevance of a multidisciplinary team approach to managing spinal cord injuries.

The fourth section includes chapters on allopathic and non-allopathic medications for managing neurological conditions, the use of phytotherapy by indigenous people in Morocco, and pharmacological modulation of toll-like receptors in brain disorders.

The editors would like to thank Author Service Manager Maja Bozicevic at IntechOpen for her fantastic work and assistance throughout the preparation of this book.

Mario Bernardo-Filho
Instituto de Biologia Roberto Alcantara Gomes and Policlínica Piquet Carneiro,
Universidade do Estado do Rio de Janeiro,
Rio de Janeiro, Brazil

Redha Taiar
Université de Reims Champagne Ardennes,
Reims, France

Danúbia da Cunha de Sá-Caputo
Instituto de Biologia Roberto Alcantara Gomes and Policlínica Piquet Carneiro,
Universidade do Estado do Rio de Janeiro; and Faculdade Bezerra de Araújo,
Rio de Janeiro, Brazil

Adérito Seixas
Escola Superior de Saúde Fernando Pessoa,
Porto, Portugal

Section 1

Introduction

Chapter 1

Introductory Chapter: Neurological Disorders - Therapy Approaches

Danúbia da Cunha de Sá-Caputo, Mario Bernardo-Filho, Adérito Seixas and Redha Taiar

1. Introduction

Neurological disorders (ND) are diseases of the central or peripheral nervous system. In other words, they affect the brain, spinal cord, cranial nerves, peripheral nerves, nerve roots, vegetative nervous system, neuro-muscular junction, and muscles. These disorders include epilepsy, Alzheimer's disease and other dementias, cerebrovascular diseases including stroke, migraine and other headaches, multiple sclerosis, Parkinson's disease, nervous system infections, brain tumors, traumatic nervous system disorders such as head injuries, and neurological disorders related to malnutrition. The result of these imbalances is that human voluntary daily life movement is affected. In fact, the achievement of the human voluntary movement seemingly simple rather it is considerably complex. As it is a very complex mechanism which allows many nerve structures to make decisional and/or reflexional choices. Then this mechanism "defines" and "controls" the movement, through the nerve impulses intended for the musculoskeletal system. It is also known that ND are the main cause of disability and the second cause of death in the world [1–4]. Some approaches and relationships about the ND are presented **Figure 1**.

The etiology of ND is very varied due to complexity of nervous system. Among the causes of ND there are: lifestyle, infections, genetics, food and/or environmental influences. Genetic, epigenetic, and various external factors, such as physical trauma, infection, and different aspects of the environmental surroundings can be involved with the initiation and the progression of the ND. Hormonal, immune, and molecular/cellular pathways impact the clinical presentation of the ND involving various systems [5]. Moreover, gut dysbiosis (microbiota dysregulation) has been associated with some neurodegenerative diseases [6]. ND can negatively influence the bone physiology favoring decrease of the bone mineral density and bone mineral content, altered bone microarchitecture, and decrease bone strength, contributing to the development of osteopenia/osteoporosis and increased of risk of fracture [5].

The neurodegeneration is presented in several ND [6]. This condition occurs when the nervous system or neuron loses its structure, function, or both, leading to progressive degeneration or the death of neurons, and well-defined associations of tissue system, resulting in clinical manifestations. Studies have been reported that the neuroinflammation precede neurodegeneration in various ND [5]. In this context,

IntechOpen

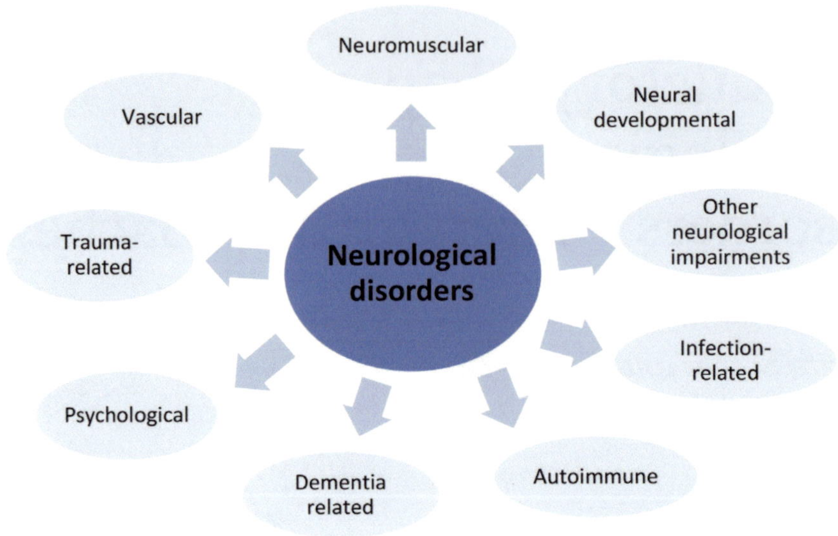

Figure 1.
APPROACHES and relationships about the neurological disorders.

appears that matrix metalloproteinases have a crucial role in the progression of ND related to neurodegeneration, although the etiology and potential causes remain widely indefinable [7].

According to the type of ND and the specific affected area, the symptoms are presented. The symptoms can be: i) complete or partial paralysis, ii) muscle weakness, iii) partial or complete loss of sensitivity, iv) convulsions, v) headache, vi) pain without apparent causes, vii) poor coordination and viii) reduced state of consciousness [8]. They can be individually observed or together. As the nervous system is strongly related of the behavior, some neurological diseases also manifest themselves with emotional or behavioral changes. In this context, the symptoms can be sudden changes in mood, or sudden outbursts of anger, depression, altered memory, hallucinations, sleep disorders, mental confusion, among others [9].

The evaluation in ND can identify signs that suggest alteration of the nervous system and can indicate the most appropriate complementary examinations to stablish an accurate diagnosis. Among the complementary exams there are: i) imaging studies [10–13] (such as Magnetic Resonance Imaging, Computed Tomography, positron emission tomography, Ultrasonography and Doppler); ii) physiological studies (such as neurophysiological examinations [14]: electroencephalogram, electroneuromyography, evoked potentials); iii) neuropsychological tests (tests that involve interviews, questionnaire applications and specific tests, with the aim of testing areas such as attention, memory, language, reasoning, and learning); iv) analysis of cerebrospinal fluid; v) blood tests (including genetic tests, research of therapeutic levels of drugs in the body, tests for specific antibodies, and general tests for numerous other diseases that can cause neurological symptoms); and vi) biopsies (of nervous tissue, skin, or muscles). The rapid and accurate diagnosis of ND allows for early treatment, improving the quality of life and the prognosis of the disease, often being the difference between life and death [15].

ND are multifactorial and can affect several areas of functionality and if left untreated, they can result in serious consequences. The evolution and the results are depending on the severity of the disease, the type of the disease, the time between onset of symptoms and treatment, among other factors. Thus, the treatment of ND can involve medication, surgeries, multidisciplinary interventions, and other types

Neurological disorder	Definition/Etiology/Prevalence	Signals and symptoms
Multiple sclerosis [17–19]	It is considered as the most prevalent chronic inflammatory disease of the central nervous system associated with inflammatory demyelination and astroglial activation, where the neuronal and axonal injury as the leading factors of disability. Young individuals (20 to 40 years old), generally, are more affected, and late-onset multiple sclerosis characterized when symptoms initiating after 50 years. About 2,500,000 individuals have multiple sclerosis in worldwide.	The symptoms are different for each person, depending on location of neural injury in the body. The most common are fatigue, vision problems, failure to control the bladder and loss of balance. The demyelinating lesions in the brain and spinal cord contributions to progressive disability, impacting negatively on the daily physical and social activities, and cognition.
Alzheimer disease [20–22]	It is the most cause of dementia (60–80% of dementia cases), with clinical presentation of progressive anterograde episodic memory impairment, affecting memory, thinking and behavior. Generally, most people with Alzheimer's are 65 and older. The early-onset Alzheimer's occur when affect individuals under the 65 years. It is the sixth leading cause of death in the United States and its worldwide prevalence is estimated in 24 million.	The early symptom is related the difficulty remembering newly learned information. The symptoms can grow severe and interfere with daily tasks, including disorientation, mood and behavior changes, confusion about events, time and place, unfounded suspicions about family, friends and professional caregivers, and difficulty speaking, swallowing, and walking.
Parkinson disease [23, 24]	It is a neurodegenerative disorder that affects dopamine-producing neurons in the substantia nigra. It is the second most common neurodegenerative disease worldwide, leading to significant physical, mental, social, and financial burden on patients and caregivers. According to the increase in age, the incidence of it increases too, however, four percent of people are diagnosed before age 50. It is estimated that more than 10 million people worldwide are living with Parkinson Disease.	The cardinal features are resting tremor, cogwheel rigidity, bradykinesia, and postural instability, often preceded by prodromal symptoms such as autonomic dysfunction appearing 5 to 20 years earlier. Generally, the symptoms develop slowly over years, differing from one person to another due to the diversity of the disease.
Cerebral palsy [25, 26]	It is a complex motor disorder at the level of the central nervous system caused by irreversible brain lesions that occur before, during or shortly after birth. It is the most common physical disability in childhood. It affects people in different ways that can compromise body movement, muscle control, muscle coordination, muscle tone, reflex, posture, and balance. Cerebral palsy is a permanent life-long, but some of these signs can improve or worsen over time. Cerebral palsy has a prevalence of 1 in 700 live births, affecting about 18 million people worldwide.	It is common the presence of reduction in the motor repertoire of gestures and a loss in the quality of movement with reduction of normal motor patterns. The postures which the child adopt and maintain, as well as their stability, is altered: the child has difficulty in both moving and staying still. The more alterations are, the more severe is the final paralysis and consequently the greater the disability.

Neurological disorder	Definition/Etiology/Prevalence	Signals and symptoms
Autism spectrum disorder [27, 28]	It is a neurodevelopmental disorder characterized by deficits in social communication and the presence of restricted interests and repetitive behaviors. This neurobiological disorder influenced by both genetic and environmental factors affecting the developing brain. It is estimated about 1.68% of United States children aged 8 years (or 1 in 59 children) are diagnosed with ASD and this estimate can be extrapolated to the worldwide.	Considering behavior, these individuals can present aggression, self-mutilation, crying, lack of eye contact, shouting, hyperactivity, involuntary imitation of someone else's movements, impulsivity, inappropriate social interaction, irritability, repetitive movements, repetition of meaningless words, meaningless repetition of the words themselves or persistent repetition of words or actions; related to the development, they can present speech delay in a child or learning disability; about cognition, can be presented lack of attention or intense interest in a limited number of things; considering psychological symptoms, they can present depression or ignores the emotions of others; in speech, they can present speech disorder or loss of speech. These individuals can also present tiptoeing, anxiety, lack of empathy, sensitivity to sound or tic.
Amyotrofic lateral sclerosis [29, 30]	It is characterized as a progressive neurodegenerative disease that affects nerve cells in the brain and the spinal cord, affecting controlling voluntary muscle movement compromising movements like chewing, walking, and talking. As this disease is progressive, the symptoms get worse over time. The prevalence is estimated in 5 per 100,000 in the United States; being about 30,000 individuals present this condition.	The common symptoms are fasciculations (muscle twitches) in the arm, leg, shoulder, or tongue, muscle cramps, tight and stiff muscles (spasticity), muscle weakness affecting an arm, a leg, neck, or diaphragm, slurred and nasal speech, difficulty chewing or swallowing
Myastenia graves [31–34]	It is an autoimmune disorder of neuromuscular transmission, characterized as an error in the transmission of nerve impulses to muscles, that promote fluctuating weakness and disabling fatigability. The prevalence is estimated in approximately 20 cases per 100,000 population, affecting twice as many women as men, however, considering older individuals, men appear are affected more often.	The mainly symptom is muscle weakness that worsens after periods of activity and improves after periods of rest. Muscles such as those that control eye and eyelid movement, facial expression, chewing, talking, and swallowing are compromised, generally, but not always. The symptoms that ca be presented are ocular myasthenia, ptosis, diplopia, dysarthria, weakness in the arms, hands, fingers, legs, and neck. The severe weakness of myasthenia gravis may cause respiratory failure.
Spinal cord injury [35, 36]	It is often the result of an unpredictable accident or violent event. This condition is frequently associated with severe clinical-neurological deficits leading to persisting physical and psychological sequela. It can be caused by: a violent attack (as a stabbing or a gunshot), diving into water that's too, shallow and hitting the bottom trauma during a car accident (as a trauma to the face, head, and neck region, back, or chest area), falling from a significant height, head, or spinal injuries (as during sporting events), and electrical accidents. It is estimated that 327 million people are affected with this condition annually	The symptoms can be related to difficulty in walking, loss of control of the bladder or bowels, inability to move the arms or legs, feelings of spreading numbness or tingling in the extremities, headache, pain, pressure, and stiffness in the back or neck area, signs of shock, unnatural positioning of the head.

Neurological disorder	Definition/Etiology/Prevalence	Signals and symptoms
Traumatic Brain Injury [37, 38]	It is characterized as a damage in the brain by an external mechanical force, leading to temporary/permanent secondary injuries. This alteration can promote impairment of cognitive, physical, and psycho-social functions with altered consciousness. The mainly mechanism responsible for neuronal damage in this condition is an increase in oxidative reactions initiated by free radicals generated by the injury. It is considered as a leading cause of mortality, morbidity, and disability worldwide, and it is estimated that 5.3 million of individuals in United States (2 percent of the population) present a disability as a result of a traumatic brain injury.	The signs and symptoms related to mild traumatic brain injuries are: physical symptoms (headache, nausea or vomiting, fatigue or drowsiness, problems with speech, dizziness or loss of balance, sensory symptoms, sensory problems - such as blurred vision, ringing in the ears, a bad taste in the mouth or changes in the ability to smell Sensitivity to light or sound; cognitive, behavioral, or mental symptoms; loss of consciousness for a few seconds to a few minutes; without loss of consciousness, but a state of being dazed, confused or disoriented; memory or concentration problems; mood changes or mood swings; feeling depressed or anxious; difficulty sleeping; sleeping more than usual. Considering moderate to severe traumatic brain injuries can be present: physical symptoms; loss of consciousness from several minutes to hours; persistent headache or headache that worsens; repeated vomiting or nausea; convulsions or seizures; dilation of one or both pupils of the eyes; clear fluids draining from the nose or ears; inability to awaken from sleep; weakness or numbness in fingers and toes; loss of coordination; cognitive or mental symptoms; profound confusion; agitation; slurred speech; coma and other disorders of consciousness.
Stroke [39, 40]	There are 3 types of strokes: ischemic stroke (when blood flow through the artery to the brain becomes blocked, such as blood clots); hemorrhagic stroke (when an artery in the brain breaks and puts too much pressure on brain cells damaging them, that can be intracerebral hemorrhage or subarachnoid hemorrhage); and transient ischemic attack (when blood flow to the brain is blocked for only a short time—usually no more than 5 minutes). The ischemic stroke corresponds to 87% of strokes. More than 795,000 individuals in the United States have a stroke, annually.	The symptoms related to this condition can be sudden numbness or weakness in the face, arm, or leg, especially on one side of the body; sudden confusion, trouble speaking, or difficulty understanding speech; sudden trouble seeing in one or both eyes; sudden trouble walking, dizziness, loss of balance, or lack of coordination, and sudden severe headache with no known cause.

Table 1.
Considerations about determined neurological disorders.

of available treatments to help the improvement of these patients. Among the physical therapies and other treatments, there are: i) movement, exercise, and physical activity therapies to improve the individual's motor capacity; ii) speech therapy, which improves the functioning of swallowing and a language; iii) occupational/cognitive therapies to stimulate functionality, working on the affected cognitive areas, such as memory, verbal and written communication, language, etc.; iv) psychotherapy for the treatment of the emotional components of the disease. Drug treatments for many ND, such as selective serotonin reuptake inhibitors, antipsychotics, anti-epilepsy drugs have independent and overlapping roles in mediating bone loss [5, 16].

In this introductory chapter, some considerations about determined ND will be presented and discussed, as indicated in **Table 1**.

2. General approaches in ND

The functional capacity and quality of life of individuals with ND can be affected in different ways according to the injured area, the extension of the injury, the time of the injury and the age of the patient. The symptoms associated differing to each ND and can be related to impairments in movements, cognition, behavior, balance, tonus, bone and spasticity among others [41, 42].

The therapeutical approaches are stablished according to the type of ND and evolution of them. These approaches can involve pharmacological and non-pharmacological interventions, neurological physical therapy, biological and molecular approaches, among other that aim to management of the ND, improving functionality, daily activities, and quality of life of these individuals [43, 44].

3. Conclusion

It is known that Neurological disorders include all diseases and dysfunctions of the central or peripheral nervous system under the same name. It is known that Hundreds of millions of people worldwide suffer from neurological disorders. It is also known that neurological conditions pose an economic burden to society. The purpose of this chapter is to summarize the impact of neurological disorders on patients' quality of life and to acknowledge their importance. This chapter will provide a better understanding of neurological disorders, assessments, prevention decisions, medical consultation, and treatments. In our present chapter, it is concluded that ND can impact the life of the individual in all aspects and the lesions are related to the area, injury, time, and age of them. The therapeutical approaches are selected according to type and evolution of ND and involves multidisciplinary treatments. These approaches seek to promote a cure or the autonomy of individual for a long time as possible with quality of life.

Author details

Danúbia da Cunha de Sá-Caputo[1,2], Mario Bernardo-Filho[1*], Adérito Seixas[3] and Redha Taiar[4]

1 Laboratório de Vibrações Mecânicas e Práticas Integrativas, Instituto de Biologia Roberto Alcantara Gomes and Policlínica Piquet Carneiro, Universidade do Estado do Rio de Janeiro, Rio de Janeiro, Brazil

2 Faculdade Bezerra de Araújo, Curso de Fisioterapia, Rio de Janeiro, RJ, Brazil

3 Escola Superior de Saúde Fernando Pessoa, Porto, Portugal

4 Université de Reims, Reims, France

*Address all correspondence to: bernardofilhom@gmail.com

References

[1] Feigin VL, Abajobir AA, Abate KH, et al. Global, regional, and national burden of neurological disorders during 1990-2015: a systematic analysis for the Global Burden of Disease Study 2015. The Lancet Neurology. 2017;16(11):877-897.

[2] Collaborators GUND. Burden of Neurological Disorders Across the US From 1990-2017: A Global Burden of Disease Study. JAMA Neurology. 2021;78(2):165-176.

[3] Chin JH, Vora N. The global burden of neurologic diseases. Neurology. 2014;83(4):349.

[4] Erkkinen MG, Kim MO, Geschwind MD. Clinical Neurology and Epidemiology of the Major Neurodegenerative Diseases. *Cold Spring Harb Perspect Biol.* 2018;10(4).

[5] Kelly RR, Sidles SJ, LaRue AC. Effects of Neurological Disorders on Bone Health. *Frontiers in Psychology.* 2020;11(3399).

[6] Gubert C, Kong G, Renoir T, Hannan AJ. Exercise, diet and stress as modulators of gut microbiota: Implications for neurodegenerative diseases. Neurobiology of Disease. 2020;134:104621.

[7] Behl T, Kaur G, Sehgal A, et al. Multifaceted Role of Matrix Metalloproteinases in Neurodegenerative Diseases: Pathophysiological and Therapeutic Perspectives. *International Journal of Molecular Sciences.* 2021;22(3).

[8] Borsook D. Neurological diseases and pain. Brain. 2012;135(2):320-344.

[9] Butler C, Zeman AZJ. Neurological syndromes which can be mistaken for psychiatric conditions. *Journal of Neurology, Neurosurgery & Psychiatry.* 2005;76(suppl 1):i31.

[10] Delin S, Bošnjak Nađ K, Martinec S, Čokolić Petrović D, Šimic Klarić A, Mejaški Bošnjak V. Prognostic value of cranial ultrasonography in comparison with magnetic resonance imaging in children with cerebral palsy: a population-based study. Acta Clin Croat. 2020;59(2):260-269.

[11] Lim M, Jassar H, Kim DJ, Nascimento TD, DaSilva AF. Differential alteration of fMRI signal variability in the ascending trigeminal somatosensory and pain modulatory pathways in migraine. The Journal of Headache and Pain. 2021;22(1):4.

[12] Michler E, Kaiser D, Eleftheriadou K, Falkenburger B, Kotzerke J, Hoberück S. Comparison of 6-[18F]FDOPA PET with Nigrosome 1 detection in patients with parkinsonism. EJNMMI Research. 2021;11(1):16.

[13] Palermo F, Pieroni N, Maugeri L, et al. X-ray Phase Contrast Tomography Serves Preclinical Investigation of Neurodegenerative Diseases. *Frontiers in Neuroscience.* 2020;14(1137).

[14] Guérit JM, Amantini A, Amodio P, et al. Consensus on the use of neurophysiological tests in the intensive care unit (ICU): Electroencephalogram (EEG), evoked potentials (EP), and electroneuromyography (ENMG). Neurophysiologie Clinique/Clinical Neurophysiology. 2009;39(2):71-83.

[15] Boersma I, Miyasaki J, Kutner J, Kluger B. Palliative care and neurology: time for a paradigm shift. Neurology. 2014;83(6):561-567.

[16] Ortuño MJ, Robinson ST, Subramanyam P, et al. Serotonin-reuptake inhibitors act centrally to cause bone loss in mice by counteracting a local anti-resorptive effect. Nature medicine. 2016;22(10):1170-1179.

[17] Momtazmanesh S, Shobeiri P, Saghazadeh A, et al. Neuronal and glial CSF biomarkers in multiple sclerosis: a systematic review and meta-analysis. Reviews in the Neurosciences. 2021.

[18] Naseri A, Nasiri E, Sahraian MA, Daneshvar S, Talebi M. Clinical Features of Late-Onset Multiple Sclerosis: a Systematic Review and Meta-analysis. Multiple Sclerosis and Related Disorders. 2021;50:102816.

[19] Marin CE, Kfouri PP, Callegaro D, et al. Patients and neurologists have different perceptions of multiple sclerosis symptoms, care and challenges. Multiple Sclerosis and Related Disorders. 2021;50:102806.

[20] Shea Y-F, Pan Y, Mak HK-F, et al. A systematic review of atypical Alzheimer's disease including behavioural and psychological symptoms. *Psychogeriatrics.* 2021;n/a(n/a).

[21] Fowler NR, Judge KS, Lucas K, et al. Feasibility and acceptability of an acceptance and commitment therapy intervention for caregivers of adults with Alzheimer's disease and related dementias. BMC Geriatrics. 2021;21(1):127.

[22] Mayeux R, Stern Y. Epidemiology of Alzheimer disease. *Cold Spring Harb Perspect Med.* 2012;2(8).

[23] Postuma RB, Berg D. Advances in markers of prodromal Parkinson disease. Nature Reviews Neurology. 2016;12(11):622-634.

[24] Muangpaisan W, Mathews A, Hori H, Seidel D. A systematic review of the worldwide prevalence and incidence of Parkinson's disease. J Med Assoc Thai. 2011;94(6):749-755.

[25] McNamara L, Scott KM, Boyd RN, Novak I. Consensus of physician behaviours to target for early diagnosis of cerebral palsy: A Delphi study. *Journal of Paediatrics and Child Health.* 2021;n/a(n/a).

[26] McMorris CA, Lake J, Dobranowski K, et al. Psychiatric disorders in adults with cerebral palsy. Research in Developmental Disabilities. 2021;111:103859.

[27] American Psychiatric Association. *Diagnostic and Statistical Manual of Mental Disorders (DSM-5®).* American Psychiatric Publishing; 2013.

[28] Hodges H, Fealko C, Soares N. Autism spectrum disorder: definition, epidemiology, causes, and clinical evaluation. Transl Pediatr. 2020;9(Suppl 1):S55-S65.

[29] Longinetti E, Fang F. Epidemiology of amyotrophic lateral sclerosis: an update of recent literature. Curr Opin Neurol. 2019;32(5):771-776.

[30] Yang T, Hou Y, Li C, et al. Risk factors for cognitive impairment in amyotrophic lateral sclerosis: a systematic review and meta-analysis. *Journal of Neurology, Neurosurgery & Psychiatry.* 2021:jnnp-2020-325701.

[31] Nalbantoglu M, Akalin MA, Gunduz A, Kiziltan M. Electro-physiological investigation for autonomic dysfunction in patients with myasthenia gravis: A prospective study. Ideggyogy Sz. 2021;74(1-2): 33-40.

[32] Hou J, Cao J, Tan P, Yu Y. Pneumocystis jiroveci pneumonia, Nocardia brasiliensis, and *Mycobacterium tuberculosis* co-infection in a myasthenia gravis patient: A case report. *Medicine.* 2021;100(1).

[33] Spillane J, Higham E, Kullmann DM. Myasthenia gravis. BMJ: British Medical Journal. 2012;345:e8497.

[34] Li Y, Arora Y, Levin K. Myasthenia gravis: newer therapies offer sustained improvement. Cleve Clin J Med. 2013;80(11):711-721.

[35] Sohn S, Kim J, Chung CK, Lee NR, Sohn MJ, Kim SH. A Nation-Wide Epidemiological Study of Newly Diagnosed Primary Spine Tumor in the Adult Korean Population, 2009-2011. J Korean Neurosurg Soc. 2017;60(2):195-204.

[36] Lo J, Chan L, Flynn S. A Systematic Review of the Incidence, Prevalence, Costs, and Activity and Work Limitations of Amputation, Osteoarthritis, Rheumatoid Arthritis, Back Pain, Multiple Sclerosis, Spinal Cord Injury, Stroke, and Traumatic Brain Injury in the United States: A 2019 Update. Archives of Physical Medicine and Rehabilitation. 2021;102(1):115-131.

[37] Kaur A, Jaiswal G, Brar J, Kumar P. Neuroprotective effect of nerolidol in traumatic brain injury associated behavioural comorbidities in rats. Toxicology Research. 2021;10(1):40-50.

[38] D. M. Sosin JESDJT. Incidence of mild and moderate brain injury in the United States, 1991. Brain Injury. 1996;10(1):47-54.

[39] Mozaffarian D, Benjamin Emelia J, Go Alan S, et al. Heart Disease and Stroke Statistics—2016 Update. Circulation. 2016;133(4):e38-e360.

[40] Esmael A, Elsherief M, Eltoukhy K. Predictive Value of the Alberta Stroke Program Early CT Score (ASPECTS) in the Outcome of the Acute Ischemic Stroke and Its Correlation with Stroke Subtypes, NIHSS, and Cognitive Impairment. Stroke Research and Treatment. 2021;2021:5935170.

[41] Nonnekes J, Goselink RJ, Růžička E, Fasano A, Nutt JG, Bloem BR. Neurological disorders of gait, balance and posture: a sign-based approach. Nature Reviews Neurology. 2018;14(3):183.

[42] Duclos H, Desgranges B, Eustache F, Laisney M. Impairment of social cognition in neurological diseases. Revue neurologique. 2018;174(4):190-198.

[43] Tamburin S, Lacerenza MR, Castelnuovo G, et al. Pharmacological and non-pharmacological strategies in the integrated treatment of pain in neurorehabilitation. Evidence and recommendations from the Italian Consensus Conference on Pain in Neurorehabilitation. European journal of physical and rehabilitation medicine. 2016;52(5):741-752.

[44] Pieramico V, Esposito R, Cesinaro S, Frazzini V, Sensi SL. Effects of non-pharmacological or pharmacological interventions on cognition and brain plasticity of aging individuals. Frontiers in systems neuroscience. 2014;8:153.

Section 2

Non-Pharmacological Interventions in Neurological Disorders

Chapter 2

Whole-Body Vibration Approaches in Neurological Disorders

Mario Bernardo-Filho, Danúbia da Cunha de Sá-Caputo, Adérito Seixas and Redha Taiar

Abstract

Bipedalism in humans is associated with an upright spine, however, this condition is not found in other animals with that skill. This may have favored the ability to harness the influence of the gravitational forces on the body. Furthermore, it is suggested that human feet have evolved to facilitate bipedal locomotion, losing an opposable digit that grasped branches in favor of a longitudinal arch that stiffens the foot and aids bipedal gait. Gait is a repetition of sequences of body segments to move the body forward while maintaining balance. The bipedal gait favors the contact of the feet of the individual with the floor. As a result, the mechanical vibration (MV) generated during walking, running or other activity with the feet are, normally, are added to the body. In these various situations, the forces would induce the production of MV with consequent transmission to the whole body of the individual and there is the generation of whole-body vibration (WBV) exercise naturally. However, when a person has a disability, this normal addition of the MV to body does not occur. This also happens with the sedentary or bedridden individual due to illness. In this case, there are the MV yielded in vibrating platforms. The exposure of the individual to the WBV leads to physiological responses at musculoskeletal, neurological, endocrinological, and vascular levels. Considering the state of the art of this theme and the previously cited scientific information, it is plausible to assume that WBV could be a useful tool to be used on the management of individuals with neurological conditions, such as in Parkinson's disease, stroke, cerebral palsy, multiple sclerosis, spinal cord injuries, spinocerebellar ataxia and Duchenne muscular dystrophy, and neuropathy (diabetes- and chemotherapy-related), among others. Indeed, improvements due to the WBV have been described regarding motor, and other impairments, in patients with neurological conditions, and these approaches will be presented in this chapter.

Keywords: neurological diseases, whole-body vibration, clinical intervention, bipedalism, gait

1. Introduction

Bipedalism in humans is associated with an upright spine, however, this condition is not found in other animals with that skill. This may have favored the ability to harness the influence of the gravitational forces on the body [1].

Moreover, Bernardo-Filho et al. [2] have suggested that the increase of the load transmitted to the body due to the bipedal movement could be associated with the evolution of human beings on our planet. Furthermore, it is suggested that human feet have evolved to facilitate bipedal locomotion, losing an opposable digit that grasped branches in favor of a longitudinal arch that stiffens the foot and aids bipedal gait [3].

The Biomechanical bipedal gait involves several steps, as it is shown in **Figures 1** and **2**. Gait action can be defined as a displacement consisting on the translation of the whole body, following rotational movements. Gait is a repetition of sequences of body segments to move the body forward while maintaining balance. Walking is a complex locomotor task that depends on the satisfactory functioning of the locomotor system at all levels. It also depends on other factors such as age, size, morphology, speed. Gait is a cyclic motor activity that alternates a supporting phase (foot in contact with the ground) and an oscillating phase (no foot contact with the ground). The locomotor cycle (stride) represents all the articular and muscular events that occur between two successive strides on the ground [4].

Biomechanically, this cycle can be divided in two phases, the support or stance phase (the limb is in contact with the ground) and the transfer phase (swing phase) called oscillation or rocking phase (the limb moves above the ground). The support phase represents 60% of the gait cycle and the swing phase 40% of the gait cycle. Whether it is for the support phase or the swing phase, several sub-phases can be described [5].

The loading phase (0 to 10% of the running cycle). This phase begins with the initial contact of the foot with the ground (0 to 2%) and is determined by the lifting of the opposite foot (first bipodal support). The role is to transfer weight to the leg during the support phase, absorb shocks and maintain walking speed while maintaining balance. The middle support phase (10 to 30% of the gait cycle). This is the first half of the unipodal support. It allows the body to move forward over the supported foot and ends when the body's center of gravity is aligned with the forefoot. The end phase (30 to 50% of the gait cycle) is the second half of the unipodal support. This phase allows the body to move forward until the opposite foot touches the ground. The pre-oscillating phase (50 to 60% of the gait cycle). This phase corresponds to the second bipodal support. The role is to propel the body forward with the transfer of weight to the leg during the support phase. The oscillation start phase (60 to 73% of the gait cycle). It corresponds to the first third of the oscillation phase and ends when the foot passes by the contralateral foot. The role of this phase and the two following phases is to allow the oscillating limb to advance without contact with the ground. The middle phase of oscillation (73 to 86% of the gait cycle) and corresponds to the second third of the oscillating phase. It ends when the tibialis is vertical. Follow, the oscillation end phase (86 to 100% of the walking cycle). This phase corresponds to the third of the oscillating phase. According to

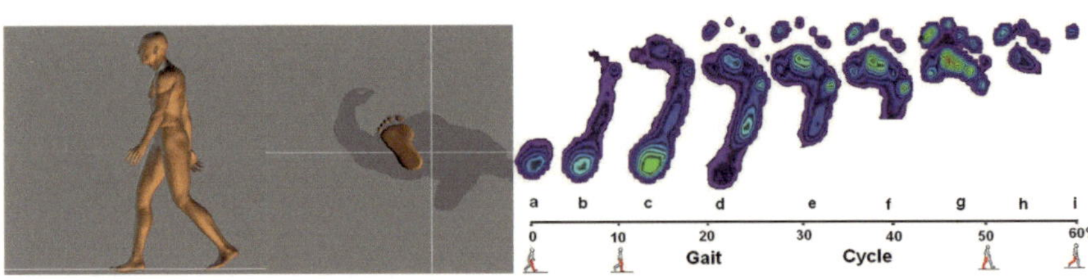

Figure 1.
Musculoskeletal complex system represented by the association of segmental movement and the complicated contact with the ground during the gait cycle. The pressure zones indicate the solicited zones during gait.

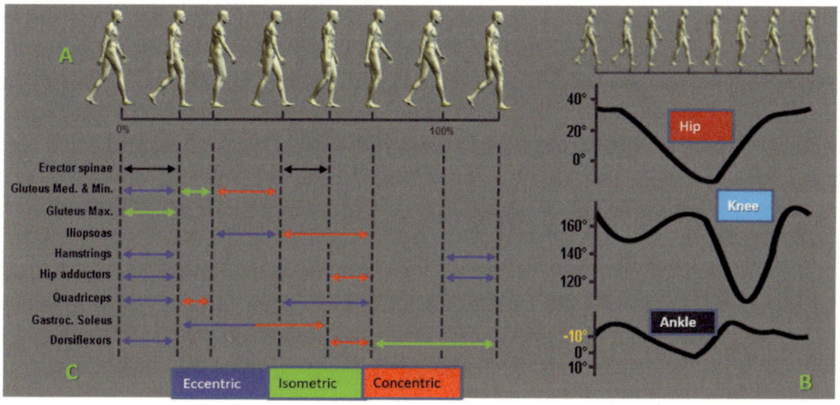

Figure 2.
Kinematics and kinetics of the normal gait.

the above description, gait movement, must have integrated and complex actions of the neuro-musculoskeletal system, and when there are dysfunctions or disabilities related to this system, the gait movement is impaired [6].

The bipedal gait favors the contact of the feet of the individual with the floor [7]. As a result, the mechanical vibration (MV) generated during walking, running or other activity with the feet are, normally, are added to the body. Cardinale and Wakeling [8], have pointed out that in the sporting activities the body interact with the external environmental and experience the action of external forces. In these various situations, the forces would induce the production of MV with consequent transmission to the whole body of the individual and there is the generation of whole-body vibration (WBV) exercise naturally. In consequence, as it would be expected, this addition of mechanical vibration has been important to the life and desirable physiological responses occur. However, when a person has a disability, this normal addition of the MV to body does not occur. This also happens with the sedentary or bedridden individual due to illness. In this case, there are the MV yielded in vibrating platforms, which types can be side alternating or vertical [9–15].

MV is a physical agent and, as a vibratory stimulus, has oscillatory and sinusoidal displacement in relation to an equilibrium position. Furthermore, the MV produced in the vibrating platform has also deterministic displacement. In consequence, it is possible to establish the biomechanical parameters, such as frequency, peak-to-peak displacement and peak acceleration to define personalized and controlled protocols that will be used in WBV exercise interventions, as it pointed out in **Table 1** [16, 17]. In a MV, the displacement between two successive points is named the cycle, without a dimension. The number of the cycles in a considered

Biomechanical	**Temporal**
Frequency	Work time
Peak-to-peak displacement	Rest time
Peak acceleration	Number of sessions and time of each session
	Number of bouts in a session and the time of each bout
	Total time of the intervention
	Week periodicity

Table 1.
Biomechanical and temporal parameters to be considered in the protocols of whole-body vibration exercises.

time is the frequency, that might express in cycle per second (s^{-1}), that is the Hertz (Hz). The displacement of the mechanical vibration has two peaks, a higher and a lower, and the vertical distance between these peaks is the peak-to-peak displacement, measured, for example, in mm. In the highest peak, it is found the maximal rate of change in velocity during a cycle, the highest acceleration, that can used to characterize the intensity of the exposition, that is the magnitude effect. As an acceleration, it is measured directly in m/s^2, or in number of times of the Earth acceleration (×g).

In the protocols involving WBV exercises, temporal parameters would be also considered, as it is also indicated in **Table 1**.

The exposure of the individual to the whole-body vibration leads to physiological responses at musculoskeletal, neurological, endocrinological, and vascular levels, as is shown in **Figure 3**.

The comprehension of these responses is important to clarify about the relevance of the whole-body vibration also to the management of individuals with several clinical conditions, such as, chronic obstructive pulmonary disease and pelvic floor, metabolic (metabolic syndrome, obesity, diabetes) and musculoskeletal disorders [2, 15, 18]. Furthermore, the individuals with neurological commitments have been also treated with interventions with whole-body vibration [11, 15, 19].

In general, related to the musculoskeletal level, whole-body vibration increases the muscle strength and the bone mineral density, endurance, and power; improves the balance and decreases the risk of falls and fractures. Furthermore, whole-body vibration also improves functionality, with an increase of the range of motion of the joints, flexibility, and improvement in gait parameters, such as gait speed [13, 15, 20–22].

Whole-body vibration induced through mechanical stimulus also induces endocrinological responses, increasing the concentration of various plasma biomarkers [23]. Furthermore, the improvement of the peripheral circulation with increase of the blood cells velocity [24–26] and peripheral microcirculation [27, 28] is relevant to facilitate the recovery of undesirable conditions related to the vascular system.

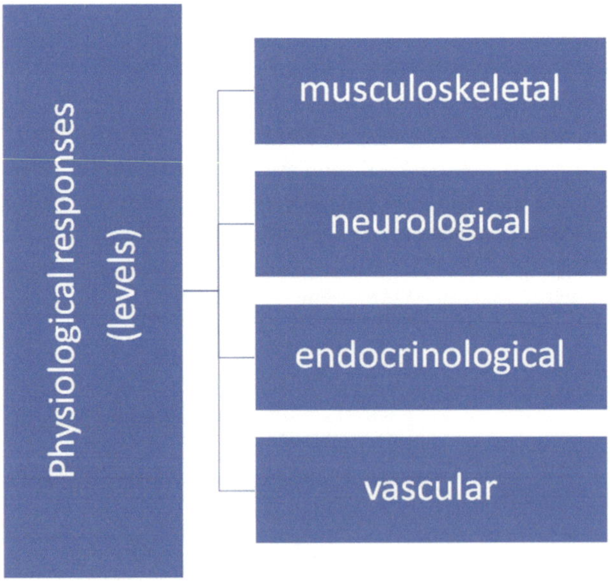

Figure 3.
Possible physiological responses to the exposure to whole-body vibration.

The purpose of this chapter was to show, considering the state of art of the theme and the scientific information, it is plausible to assume that whole-body vibration could be a useful tool to be used on the management of individuals with neurological conditions, such as in Parkinson's disease, stroke, cerebral palsy, multiple sclerosis, spinal cord injuries, spinocerebellar ataxia and Duchenne muscular dystrophy, and neuropathy (diabetes- and chemotherapy-related), among others. Indeed, improvements due to the whole-body vibration have been described regarding motor, and other impairments, in patients with neurological conditions [11, 29].

Considering the scientific information, accessed in relevant databases (PubMed, EMBASE, and SCOPUS), about the use of whole-body vibration on the management of individuals with neurological diseases, some publications were selected and used in this chapter.

2. Whole-body vibration exercise in stroke individuals

Stroke is defined as an event that blood supply to part of your brain is reduced or interrupted, leading to brain tissue from getting oxygen and nutrients. In this situation the brain cells can die in minutes. This condition needs an early action to reduce brain damage and other complications [30].

There are three types of strokes: i) ischemic stroke, referring to a block of blood flow through the artery to the brain, such as blood clots; ii) hemorrhagic stroke, characterizing a damage of the artery in the brain and pressure on brain cells, favoring the intracerebral hemorrhage or the subarachnoid hemorrhage; and iii) transient ischemic attack, that occurs when blood flow to the brain is blocked for only a short time (usually no more than 5 minutes) [31].

The ischemic stroke corresponds to 87% of strokes. More than 795,000 individuals in the United States have a stroke, annually. The general symptoms related to stroke are: sudden numbness or weakness in the face, arm, or leg, especially on one side of the body; sudden confusion, trouble speaking, or difficulty understanding speech; sudden trouble seeing in one or both eyes; sudden trouble walking, dizziness, loss of balance, or lack of coordination, and sudden severe headache with no known cause [32].

The WBV has been used in the management of stroke individuals and studies have reported improvement in functional mobility, muscle strength, spasticity. The vibration type used was vertical and side-alternating, the vibration amplitude from 1 to 4 mm, the mechanical vibration frequency from 5 to 40 Hz, the duration of each bout from 30 seconds to 2.5 minutes, and the duration of WBV protocol from 4 to 12 weeks [33–36].

3. Whole-body vibration exercise in cerebral palsy individuals

Cerebral palsy is a motor disorder at the level of the central nervous system caused by irreversible brain lesions that occur before, during or shortly after birth. Cerebral palsy has a prevalence of 1 in 700 live births, affecting about 18 million people worldwidev [37]. The individuals can present compromising of body movement, muscle control, muscle coordination, muscle tone, reflex, posture, balance, cognitive impairment, or seizures. Some symptoms of cerebral palsy are permanent life-long, but some of them can improve or worsen over time. It is common the presence of reduction in the motor repertoire of gestures and a loss in the quality of movement with reduction of normal motor patterns, alterations in posture and in stability. More alterations promote greater disability. Motor effects of cerebral palsy varied by the individual and can be pyramidal/spastic or extrapyramidal/non-spastic [38–40].

These children present difficulty to achieve and maintain an upright position in a severe cerebral palsy. As the dynamic weight bearing is unavailable, there are a predisposition of them to reduce bone mineral density and development of osteoporosis. In consequence, they can present more prone to muscle weakness, which contributes to pain, deformity and functional loss [41, 42].

Studies have reported that whole body vibration can improve spasticity, muscle strength and coordination in cerebral palsy individuals. Considering the biomechanical parameters, the WBV exercise was performed using a side-alternating or vertical platform, frequency from 5 to 35 Hz, working time from 45 seconds to 3 minutes, from 8 weeks to 6 months [19, 43–45].

4. Whole-body vibration exercise in spinal cord injury individuals

Spinal cord injury can be present because of an unpredictable accident or violent event and it is estimated that 327 million people are affected with this condition annually [46, 47]. Frequently is related to clinical-neurological deficits leading to persisting physical and psychological sequela. Spinal cordy injury can be present due: i) a violent attack, as a stabbing or a gunshot; ii) diving into water that is too, shallow and hitting the bottom; iii) trauma during a car accident, as a trauma to the face, head, and neck region, back, or chest area; iv) falling from a significant height, head or spinal injuries, as during sporting events; and v) electrical accidents [46, 47].

The symptoms can be i) difficult to walking; ii) loss of control of the bladder or bowels; iii) inability to move the arms or legs; iv) feelings of spreading numbness or tingling in the extremities; v) headache; vi) pain, pressure, and stiffness in the back or neck area; vii) signs of shock; and viii) unnatural positioning of the head [46, 47].

WBV have been used to improve spasticity, balance and walking ability in individuals [48], peripheral arterial properties [49] and walking function [50]. The protocol used in these studies involved a side-alternating platform, working time from 30 seconds to 1 minute, frequency from 8 Hz to 50 Hz, amplitude from 2 to 5 mm. The postures varied from squat position to seated in a chair with foot on the base of the platform.

5. Whole-body vibration exercise in patients with diabetic neuropathy

Nearly 15–20 million people in the United States have some type of neuropathy [51], a nerve injury affecting mostly the nerves that innervate the body extremities, in a "glove and stocking" distribution.

Hyperglycaemia, or raised blood sugar, in uncontrolled diabetes leads to serious damage to multiple body's systems over time, especially the nerves and blood vessels. Therefore, neuropathy is a common complication of diabetes, affecting up to 50% of patients with type 1 and type 2 diabetes [52, 53]. In many cases, the involvement is especially in small nerve fibers of the lower and upper limbs, with symptoms such as numbness, tingling, burning, and pain occurring first, but medium and large nerve fibers may also be affected. As disease progresses, motor symptoms such as muscle weakness in distal and then in more proximal areas, and autonomic symptoms, later on the disease course, appear (e.g. dry eyes, dry mouth, orthostatic dizziness, constipation, bladder incontinence, sexual dysfunction) [54, 55].

Study	WBV type	WBV frequency and peak-to-peak displacement, or magnitude	Other aspects
Lee et al. [56]	Side alternating	15–30 Hz, 1–3 mm	3×3-min bouts, 3 times/week for 6 weeks
Yoosefinejad et al. [57]	Vertical	30 Hz, 2 mm	30s-1 min bouts, twice/week for 6 weeks
Jamal et al. [58]	Unknown	12 Hz, 5 mm	4×3 min bouts, 3 times/week for 6 weeks
Kessler et al. [59]	Unknown	25 Hz, 0.5–1.0 g	4×3 min bouts, 3 times/week for 6 weeks

Table 2.
WBV intervention characteristics of the studies including people with diabetic neuropathy.

Results from high level of evidence primary studies position WBV as an effective intervention for people with diabetic neuropathy. Studies have reported positive effects of WBV on balance and postural control [56–58], pain [58, 59], other neuropathy signs and symptoms [58] and quality of life [58]. The characteristics of the WBV interventions are summarized in **Table 2**.

6. Whole-body vibration exercise in patients with chemotherapy-induced neuropathy

Cancer represents one of the main causes of morbidity and mortality worldwide [60]. Hopefully, the number of cancer survivors is increasing progressively due to the increasing ability to early detect and treat the conditions.

Chemotherapy-induced neuropathy (CIN) is a common side effect of cancer treatment with chemotherapy, with 68.1% of patients suffering from CIN in the first month after chemotherapy [61], 60% after 3 months and 30% after 6 months. The condition may express as sensoric and/or motor, and sometimes also autonomic dysfunction, leading to important limitations in activities of daily life [62, 63]. As other types of neuropathy CIN heavily impairs physical fitness due to the severe consequences of loss of peripheral somatosensory information on balance and locomotion [64, 65].

The relevance of WBV exercise in the management of cancer therapy-related morbidities has been addressed before [66], specifically its implications for cancer survivors suffering from CIN [67]. Evidence from high level of evidence primary studies suggest WBV to be a potentially effective intervention for cancer survivors with CIN. However, only two high level of evidence primary studies have analyzed

Study	WBV type	WBV frequency and peak-to-peak displacement, or magnitude	Other aspects
Schönsteiner et al. [62]	Side alternating	9–23 Hz, peak-to-peak displacement or magnitude not reported	18 minutes/session, 15 training sessions within 15 weeks
Streckmann et al. [68]	Side alternating	18–35 Hz, 2–4 mm	4×30s-1 min bouts, twice/week for 6 weeks

Table 3.
WBV intervention characteristics of the studies including people with CIN.

the effectiveness of WBV in this population, suggesting that WBV could prove useful to reduce pain [68], sensory ability and strength and function [62]. These information are pointed out in **Table 3**.

Although evidence of the relevance of WBV in people with neuropathy (diabetes- and chemotherapy-related) arises from high level of evidence studies, evidence from high methodological quality studies is on demand, considering some methodological issues in the studies. Therefore, high quality studies are needed to strengthen the existing body of knowledge regarding the effectiveness of WBV in people with neuropathy.

7. Whole-body vibration exercise in patients with Parkinson's disease

Neurodegenerative disorders have an high impact for both individuals and society [69] and Parkinson's disease (PD) is among this type of conditions.

PD is a slowly progressive neurodegenerative disorder, which affects nearly 1 million north Americans [70, 71]. Apart from the classic motor symptoms, such as rigidity, bradykinesia, resting tremor and postural instability, usually associated with nigrostriatal system degeneration, other non-motor symptoms, with more complex etiology, including neuroendocrine and metabolic disturbances are present [72, 73].

The burden of PD to society, payers, patients, and health professionals is high and interventions to reduce PD incidence, delay disease progression, and alleviate the disease impact, may reduce the burden of the condition [71].

The benefits of WBV in this population has proven conflicting, with studies reporting greater effects in the WBV group and studies reporting a lack of real benefit when comparing with control groups.

Two studies [74, 75] compared the acute effects of a 1-session WBV program at different vibration frequencies on balance, gait or flexibility parameters in patients with PD. One of the studies [75] suggested that higher frequencies seem to produce more effective results but only reported significant effects in flexibility after a WBV session, when compared with the control group, and the other [74] showed that none of the vibration frequencies had better results than the placebo group.

Other studies have compared the benefits of a WBV program, over several weeks, with placebo [76, 77], with an aerobic exercise program [78], conventional balance training [79] and conventional therapy and combined (conventional + WBV) therapy [80]. When compared to placebo, one study [76] reported no advantage of WBV but the other study [77] reported significantly better results in the WBV group regarding balance and gait parameters. When compared to an aerobic exercise program, the oxygen consumption during exercise was similar and the WBV group did not required a long time of recovery and led to less feeling of fatigue. When compared to conventional balance training the results were positive in both groups, however, posturography parameters only improved in the WBV group. Similarly, when compared to conventional therapy, both groups evidenced an improvement in balance. The combined therapy group (conventional + WBV) achieved significantly better results than the conventional therapy group, but not the WBV group, suggesting that WBV could be a useful co-adjuvant intervention to increase balance in PD patients. These information are indicated in **Table 4**.

WBV seems to be a promising intervention in PD, as an independent or co-adjuvant modality, but the existing result heterogeneity does not allow a confident recommendation. More good quality, placebo controlled, studies are needed to establish the clinical effectiveness of WBV in improving functional parameters in people with PD.

Study	WBV type	WBV frequency and peak-to-peak displacement, or magnitude	Other aspects
Chouza et al. [74]	Side alternating	3, 6 or 9 Hz, 13 mm	5× 1 min bouts, 1 session
Dincher et al. [75]	Side alternating	6, 12 or 18 Hz, 4 mm	5× 1 min bouts, 1 session
Arias et al. [76]	Side alternating	6 Hz, 13 mm	5× 1 min bouts, 12 sessions/5 weeks
Gaßner et al. [77]	Unknown	6 Hz, 3 mm	5× 1 min bouts, 12 sessions/5 weeks
Corbianco et al. [78]	Side alternating	26 Hz, 4 mm	20× 1 min bouts, 4 sessions/weeks for 4 weeks
Ebersbach et al. [79]	Side alternating	25 Hz, peak-to-peak displacement or magnitude not reported	15 min/session, 2 sessions/day, 5 days/week for 3 weeks
Guadarrama-Molina et al. [80]	Vertical	20 Hz, 2 mm	8× 20 sec bouts, 20 sessions, 3 sessions/week

Table 4.
WBV intervention characteristics of the studies including people with PD.

8. Summary

Whole-body vibration exercise is an exercise modality that induces musculo-skeletal, endocrinological, vascular and neurologic responses, which are relevant in the context of neurological conditions. This intervention proved to be promising for people with multiple neurological conditions and its results have been discussed for people with stroke, cerebral palsy, spinal cord injury, neuropathy (diabetes- and chemotherapy-related) and Parkinson's disease.

Author details

Mario Bernardo-Filho[1*], Danúbia da Cunha de Sá-Caputo[1,2], Adérito Seixas[3] and Redha Taiar[4]

1 Laboratório de Vibrações Mecânicas e Práticas Integrativas, Instituto de Biologia Roberto Alcantara Gomes and Policlínica Piquet Carneiro, Universidade do Estado do Rio de Janeiro, Rio de Janeiro, Brazil

2 Faculdade Bezerra de Araújo, Curso de Fisioterapia, Rio de Janeiro, RJ, Brazil

3 Universidade Fernando Pessoa, Porto, Portugal

4 Université de Reims, Reims, France

*Address all correspondence to: bernardofilhom@gmail.com

References

[1] Leisman G, Moustafa AA, Shafir T. Thinking, walking, talking: integratory motor and cognitive brain function. Frontiers in public health. 2016;4:94.

[2] Bernardo-Filho M, Bemben D, Stark C, Taiar R. Biological consequences of exposure to mechanical vibration. In: SAGE Publications Sage CA: Los Angeles, CA; 2018.

[3] Farris DJ, Kelly LA, Cresswell AG, Lichtwark GA. The functional importance of human foot muscles for bipedal locomotion. Proceedings of the National Academy of Sciences. 2019;116(5):1645-1650.

[4] Agnesina G, Taïar R. LifeMOD modelling of a complete human body: a walk with a right knee varus and valgus movement. *Journal of Biomechanics.* 2006;39(Supplement 1):S54.

[5] Perin J, Agnesina G, Taiar R, Toshev Y. Analysis of the plantar foot pressure during walking: VFE position and VRI position. *Journal of Biomechanics.* 2006;39(Supplement 1): S552-S553.

[6] Taiar R, Fogarassy P, Boyer F, Lodini A. Knee joint distribution: 3D finite element analysis. Series on Biomechanics. 2010;25(3-4):3-11.

[7] Fourchet F, Kelly L, Horobeanu C, Loepelt H, Taiar R, Millet GP. Comparison of plantar pressure distribution in adolescent runners at low vs. high running velocity. Gait & Posture. 2012;35(4):685-687.

[8] Cardinale M, Wakeling J. Whole body vibration exercise: are vibrations good for you? British journal of sports medicine. 2005;39(9):585-589.

[9] Sañudo B, Seixas A, Gloeckl R, et al. Potential Application of Whole Body Vibration Exercise for Improving the Clinical Conditions of COVID-19 Infected Individuals: A Narrative Review from the World Association of Vibration Exercise Experts (WAVex) Panel. International Journal of Environmental Research and Public Health. 2020;17(10):3650.

[10] Wollersheim T, Haas K, Wolf S, et al. Whole-body vibration to prevent intensive care unit-acquired weakness: safety, feasibility, and metabolic response. Critical Care. 2017;21(1):9.

[11] Alashram AR, Padua E, Annino G. Effects of Whole-Body Vibration on Motor Impairments in Patients With Neurological Disorders: A Systematic Review. *American Journal of Physical Medicine & Rehabilitation.* 2019;98(12).

[12] Gimigliano F. Is whole body vibration exercise training effective and safe in fibromyalgia patients? A Cochrane Review summary with commentary. Journal of musculoskeletal & neuronal interactions. 2019;19(2):133-135.

[13] Cochrane DJ. The potential neural mechanisms of acute indirect vibration. J Sports Sci Med. 2011;10(1):19-30.

[14] Alter P, Boeselt T, Nell C, Spielmanns M, Kenn K, Koczulla AR. Feasibility and safety of whole-body vibration therapy in intensive care patients. Critical Care. 2017;21(1):1-2.

[15] Rittweger J. Vibration as an exercise modality: how it may work, and what its potential might be. European Journal of Applied Physiology. 2010;108(5):877-904.

[16] Rauch F, Sievanen H, Boonen S, et al. Reporting whole-body vibration intervention studies: recommendations of the International Society of Musculoskeletal and Neuronal

Interactions. Journal of musculoskeletal & neuronal interactions. 2010;10.

[17] Wuestefeld A, Fuermaier ABM, Bernardo-Filho M, et al. Towards reporting guidelines of research using whole-body vibration as training or treatment regimen in human subjects—A Delphi consensus study. PLOS ONE. 2020;15(7):e0235905.

[18] Guedes-Aguiar EdO, de Sá-Caputo DdC, Moreira-Marconi E, et al. Effect of whole-body vibration exercise in the pelvic floor muscles of healthy and unhealthy individuals: a narrative review. Transl Androl Urol. 2019;8(4):395-404.

[19] Sá-Caputo DC, Costa-Cavalcanti R, Carvalho-Lima RP, et al. Systematic review of whole body vibration exercises in the treatment of cerebral palsy: Brief report. Developmental Neurorehabilitation. 2016;19(5):327-333.

[20] Paiva P, Figueiredo C, Reis-Silva A, et al. Acute and cumulative effects with whole-body vibration exercises using 2 biomechanical conditions on the flexibility and rating of perceived exertion in individuals with metabolic syndrome: a randomized clinical trial pilot study. Dose-Response. 2019;17(4):1559325819886495.

[21] Oliveira MP, Menzel H, Cochrane DJ, et al. Individual responses to different vibration frequencies identified by electromyography and dynamometry in different types of vibration application. Journal of strength and conditioning research. 2019.

[22] Marín PJ, Hazell TJ, García-Gutiérrez MT, Cochrane DJ. Acute unilateral leg vibration exercise improves contralateral neuromuscular performance. J Musculoskelet Neuronal Interact. 2014;14(1):58-67.

[23] Moreira-Marconi E, de Sá-Caputo DdC, Sartorio A, Bernardo-Filho M. Hormonal Responses to Vibration Therapy. In: *Manual of Vibration Exercise and Vibration Therapy.* Springer; 2020:169-184.

[24] Betik AC, Parker L, Kaur G, Wadley GD, Keske MA. Whole-Body Vibration Stimulates Microvascular Blood Flow in Skeletal Muscle. *Medicine and Science in Sports and Exercise.* 2020.

[25] Aoyama A, Yamaoka-Tojo M, Obara S, et al. Acute Effects of Whole-Body Vibration Training on Endothelial Function and Cardiovascular Response in Elderly Patients with Cardiovascular Disease A Single-Arm Pilot Study. International heart journal. 2019:18-592.

[26] Gomes-Neto M, de Sá-Caputo DdC, Paineiras-Domingos LL, et al. Effects of whole-body vibration in older adult patients with type 2 diabetes mellitus: A systematic review and meta-analysis. *Canadian journal of diabetes.* 2019;43(7):524-529. e522.

[27] Seixas A, Silva A, Gabriel J, Vardasca R. The Effect of Whole-body Vibration in the Skin Temperature of Lower Extremities in Healthy Subjects. Thermology International. 2012;22(3):59-66.

[28] Moreira-Marconi E, Moura-Fernandes MC, Lopes-Souza P, et al. Evaluation of the temperature of posterior lower limbs skin during the whole body vibration measured by infrared thermography: Cross-sectional study analysis using linear mixed effect model. PLOS ONE. 2019;14(3):e0212512.

[29] Pozo-Cruz Bd, Adsuar JC, Parraca JA, Pozo-Cruz Jd, Olivares PR, Gusi N. Using Whole-Body Vibration Training in Patients Affected with Common Neurological Diseases: A Systematic Literature Review. The Journal of Alternative and

Complementary Medicine. 2012;18(1):29-41.

[30] Ovbiagele B, Nguyen-Huynh MN. Stroke Epidemiology: Advancing Our Understanding of Disease Mechanism and Therapy. Neurotherapeutics. 2011;8(3):319.

[31] Esmael A, Elsherief M, Eltoukhy K. Predictive Value of the Alberta Stroke Program Early CT Score (ASPECTS) in the Outcome of the Acute Ischemic Stroke and Its Correlation with Stroke Subtypes, NIHSS, and Cognitive Impairment. Stroke Research and Treatment. 2021;2021:5935170.

[32] Mozaffarian D, Benjamin Emelia J, Go Alan S, et al. Heart Disease and Stroke Statistics—2016 Update. Circulation. 2016;133(4):e38-e360.

[33] Liao LR, Ng GY, Jones AY, Huang MZ, Pang MY. Whole-Body Vibration Intensities in Chronic Stroke: A Randomized Controlled Trial. Med Sci Sports Exerc. 2016;48(7):1227-1238.

[34] Alp A, Efe B, Adalı M, et al. The Impact of Whole Body Vibration Therapy on Spasticity and Disability of the Patients with Poststroke Hemiplegia. Rehabilitation Research and Practice. 2018;2018:8637573.

[35] Marín PJ, Ferrero CM, Menéndez H, Martín J, Herrero AJ. Effects of Whole-Body Vibration on Muscle Architecture, Muscle Strength, and Balance in Stroke Patients: A Randomized Controlled Trial. *American Journal of Physical Medicine & Rehabilitation*. 2013;92(10).

[36] Miyara K, Kawamura K, Matsumoto S, et al. Acute changes in cortical activation during active ankle movement after whole-body vibration for spasticity in hemiplegic legs of stroke patients: a functional near-infrared spectroscopy study. Topics in Stroke Rehabilitation. 2020;27(1):67-74.

[37] McMorris CA, Lake J, Dobranowski K, et al. Psychiatric disorders in adults with cerebral palsy. Research in Developmental Disabilities. 2021;111:103859.

[38] McNamara L, Scott KM, Boyd RN, Novak I. Consensus of physician behaviours to target for early diagnosis of cerebral palsy: A Delphi study. *Journal of Paediatrics and Child Health*. 2021;n/a(n/a).

[39] McIntyre S, Morgan C, Walker K, Novak I. Cerebral Palsy—Don't Delay. Developmental Disabilities Research Reviews. 2011;17(2):114-129.

[40] Mockford M, Caulton JM. The Pathophysiological Basis of Weakness in Children With Cerebral Palsy. *Pediatric Physical Therapy*. 2010;22(2).

[41] Dalén Y, Sääf M, Nyrén S, Mattsson E, Haglund-Åkerlind Y, Klefbeck B. Observations of four children with severe cerebral palsy using a novel dynamic platform. A case report. Advances in Physiotherapy. 2012;14(3):132-139.

[42] Kilpinen-Loisa P, Paasio T, Soiva M, et al. Low bone mass in patients with motor disability: prevalence and risk factors in 59 Finnish children. Developmental Medicine & Child Neurology. 2010;52(3):276-282.

[43] Lee B-K, Chon S-C. Effect of whole body vibration training on mobility in children with cerebral palsy: a randomized controlled experimenter-blinded study. Clinical Rehabilitation. 2013;27(7):599-607.

[44] Unger M, Jelsma J, Stark C. Effect of a trunk-targeted intervention using vibration on posture and gait in children with spastic type cerebral palsy: A randomized control trial. Developmental Neurorehabilitation. 2013;16(2):79-88.

[45] Wren TAL, Lee DC, Hara R, et al. Effect of high-frequency, low-magnitude vibration on bone and muscle in children with cerebral palsy. J Pediatr Orthop. 2010;30(7):732-738.

[46] Sohn S, Kim J, Chung CK, Lee NR, Sohn MJ, Kim SH. A Nation-Wide Epidemiological Study of Newly Diagnosed Primary Spine Tumor in the Adult Korean Population, 2009-2011. J Korean Neurosurg Soc. 2017;60(2):195-204.

[47] Lo J, Chan L, Flynn S. A Systematic Review of the Incidence, Prevalence, Costs, and Activity and Work Limitations of Amputation, Osteoarthritis, Rheumatoid Arthritis, Back Pain, Multiple Sclerosis, Spinal Cord Injury, Stroke, and Traumatic Brain Injury in the United States: A 2019 Update. Archives of Physical Medicine and Rehabilitation. 2021;102(1):115-131.

[48] In T, Jung K, Lee M-G, Cho H-y. Whole-body vibration improves ankle spasticity, balance, and walking ability in individuals with incomplete cervical spinal cord injury. NeuroRehabilitation. 2018;42:491-497.

[49] Menéndez H, Ferrero C, Martín-Hernández J, Figueroa A, Marín PJ, Herrero AJ. Acute effects of simultaneous electromyostimulation and vibration on leg blood flow in spinal cord injury. Spinal Cord. 2016;54(5):383-389.

[50] Estes S, Iddings JA, Ray S, Kirk-Sanchez NJ, Field-Fote EC. Comparison of Single-Session Dose Response Effects of Whole Body Vibration on Spasticity and Walking Speed in Persons with Spinal Cord Injury. Neurotherapeutics. 2018;15(3):684-696.

[51] Gregg EW, Gu Q, Williams D, et al. Prevalence of lower extremity diseases associated with normal glucose levels, impaired fasting glucose, and diabetes among US adults aged 40 or older. Diabetes research and clinical practice. 2007;77(3):485-488.

[52] Young M, Boulton A, MacLeod A, Williams D, Sonksen P. A multicentre study of the prevalence of diabetic peripheral neuropathy in the United Kingdom hospital clinic population. Diabetologia. 1993;36(2):150-154.

[53] Iqbal Z, Azmi S, Yadav R, et al. Diabetic peripheral neuropathy: epidemiology, diagnosis, and pharmacotherapy. Clinical therapeutics. 2018;40(6):828-849.

[54] Callaghan BC, Gallagher G, Fridman V, Feldman EL. Diabetic neuropathy: what does the future hold? Diabetologia. 2020;63(5):891-897.

[55] Alam U. Diabetic Neuropathy Collection: Introduction to Diabetic Neuropathy. In: Springer; 2020.

[56] Lee K, Lee S, Song C. Whole-body vibration training improves balance, muscle strength and glycosylated hemoglobin in elderly patients with diabetic neuropathy. The Tohoku journal of experimental medicine. 2013;231(4):305-314.

[57] Yoosefinejad AK, Shadmehr A, Olyaei G, Talebian S, Bagheri H, Mohajeri-Tehrani MR. Short-term effects of the whole-body vibration on the balance and muscle strength of type 2 diabetic patients with peripheral neuropathy: a quasi-randomized-controlled trial study. Journal of Diabetes & Metabolic Disorders. 2015;14(1):1-8.

[58] Jamal A, Ahmad I, Ahamed N, Azharuddin M, Alam F, Hussain ME. Whole body vibration showed beneficial effect on pain, balance measures and quality of life in painful diabetic peripheral neuropathy: a randomized controlled trial. Journal of Diabetes & Metabolic Disorders. 2019:1-9.

[59] Kessler NJ, Lockard MM, Fischer J. Whole body vibration improves symptoms of diabetic peripheral neuropathy. Journal of Bodywork and Movement Therapies. 2020;24(2):1-3.

[60] Bray F, Ferlay J, Soerjomataram I, Siegel RL, Torre LA, Jemal A. Global cancer statistics 2018: GLOBOCAN estimates of incidence and mortality worldwide for 36 cancers in 185 countries. CA: a cancer journal for clinicians. 2018;68(6):394-424.

[61] Seretny M, Currie GL, Sena ES, et al. Incidence, prevalence, and predictors of chemotherapy-induced peripheral neuropathy: a systematic review and meta-analysis. *PAIN®*. 2014;155(12):2461-2470.

[62] Schönsteiner SS, Mißbach HB, Benner A, et al. A randomized exploratory phase 2 study in patients with chemotherapy-related peripheral neuropathy evaluating whole-body vibration training as adjunct to an integrated program including massage, passive mobilization and physical exercises. Experimental hematology & oncology. 2017;6(1):1-11.

[63] von Hehn CA, Baron R, Woolf CJ. Deconstructing the neuropathic pain phenotype to reveal neural mechanisms. Neuron. 2012;73(4):638-652.

[64] Cavanagh P, Derr J, Ulbrecht J, Maser R, Orchard T. Problems with gait and posture in neuropathic patients with insulin-dependent diabetes mellitus. Diabetic Medicine. 1992;9(5):469-474.

[65] Zedan AH, Hansen TF, Svenningsen ÅF, Vilholm OJ. Oxaliplatin-induced neuropathy in colorectal cancer: many questions with few answers. Clinical colorectal cancer. 2014;13(2):73-80.

[66] Lopes-Souza P, Dionello CF, da Cunha Sá-Caputo D, et al. Whole body vibration exercise in the management of cancer therapy-related morbidities: A systematic review. Drug discoveries & therapeutics. 2018;12(4):239-247.

[67] Verhulst AL, Savelberg HH, Vreugdenhil G, Mischi M, Schep G. Whole-body vibration as a modality for the rehabilitation of peripheral neuropathies: implications for cancer survivors suffering from chemotherapy-induced peripheral neuropathy. *Oncology reviews.* 2015;9(1).

[68] Streckmann F, Lehmann H, Balke M, et al. Sensorimotor training and whole-body vibration training have the potential to reduce motor and sensory symptoms of chemotherapy-induced peripheral neuropathy—a randomized controlled pilot trial. Supportive Care in Cancer. 2019;27(7):2471-2478.

[69] Zahra W, Rai SN, Birla H, et al. The global economic impact of neurodegenerative diseases: Opportunities and challenges. Bioeconomy for Sustainable Development. 2020:333-345.

[70] Marras C, Beck J, Bower J, et al. Prevalence of Parkinson's disease across North America. NPJ Parkinson's disease. 2018;4(1):1-7.

[71] Yang W, Hamilton JL, Kopil C, et al. Current and projected future economic burden of Parkinson's disease in the US. *npj Parkinson's Disease.* 2020;6(1):1-9.

[72] DeMaagd G, Philip A. Parkinson's disease and its management: part 1: disease entity, risk factors, pathophysiology, clinical presentation, and diagnosis. Pharmacy and therapeutics. 2015;40(8):504.

[73] De Pablo-Fernández E, Breen DP, Bouloux PM, Barker RA, Foltynie T, Warner TT. Neuroendocrine abnormalities in Parkinson's disease.

Journal of Neurology, Neurosurgery & Psychiatry. 2017;88(2):176-185.

[74] Chouza M, Arias P, Viñas S, Cudeiro J. Acute effects of whole-body vibration at 3, 6, and 9 hz on balance and gait in patients with Parkinson's disease. Movement Disorders. 2011;26(5):920-921.

[75] Dincher A, Becker P, Wydra G. Effect of whole-body vibration on freezing and flexibility in Parkinson's disease—a pilot study. Neurological Sciences. 2020:1-7.

[76] Arias P, Chouza M, Vivas J, Cudeiro J. Effect of whole body vibration in Parkinson's disease: a controlled study. Movement disorders: official journal of the Movement Disorder Society. 2009;24(6):891-898.

[77] Gaßner H, Janzen A, Schwirtz A, Jansen P. Random whole body vibration over 5 weeks leads to effects similar to placebo: a controlled study in Parkinson's disease. Parkinson's disease. 2014;2014.

[78] Corbianco S, Cavallini G, Baldereschi G, et al. Whole body vibration and treadmill training in Parkinson's disease rehabilitation: Effects on energy cost and recovery phases. Neurological Sciences. 2018;39(12):2159-2168.

[79] Ebersbach G, Edler D, Kaufhold O, Wissel J. Whole body vibration versus conventional physiotherapy to improve balance and gait in Parkinson's disease. Archives of physical medicine and rehabilitation. 2008;89(3):399-403.

[80] Guadarrama-Molina E, Barrón-Gámez CE, Estrada-Bellmann I, et al. Comparison of the effect of whole-body vibration therapy versus conventional therapy on functional balance of patients with Parkinson's disease: adding a mixed group. Acta Neurologica Belgica. 2020:1-8.

Chapter 3

Impact of Biofeedback Interventions on Driving Performance in Individuals with Persistent Post-Concussive Symptoms

Marquise M. Bonn, Liliana Alvarez, James W.G. Thompson and James P. Dickey

Abstract

Low resolution electromagnetic tomography (LoRETA) neurofeedback and heart rate variability (HRV) biofeedback may improve driving ability by enhancing attention, impulse control, and peripheral vision, and reducing stress. However, it is unclear whether combined LoRETA neurofeedback and HRV biofeedback can improve driving performance for individuals experiencing persistent post-concussive symptoms (PPCS). In this study, seven individuals with PPCS completed an eight-week LoRETA neurofeedback and HRV biofeedback intervention. Changes in participants' simulated driving performance and self-reported symptoms were measured and compared to two control groups: individuals with PPCS (n = 9), and healthy control participants (n = 8). Individuals in the intervention and PPCS control groups reported reduced PPCS severity ($p < .05$) compared to healthy control participants. Interestingly, individuals in the intervention group responded variably. These results indicate that more research is necessary to identify the subgroup of individuals that respond to LoRETA neurofeedback and HRV biofeedback and confirm these preliminary results.

Keywords: concussion, persistent post-concussion symptoms, neurofeedback, biofeedback, driving

1. Introduction

A concussion is defined as a mild traumatic brain injury induced by biomechanical forces, which results in an array of signs and symptoms that can include somatic, cognitive, behavioral or emotional changes, sleep disturbances and/or balance problems [1]. Most concussions resolve spontaneously, but some studies indicate that as many as 43% of individuals continue to experience persistent and disabling impairments months after their injury [2]. Persistent post-concussive symptoms (PPCS) refer to the lack of clinical recovery within 10–14 days for adults, and within four weeks for children [1]. As described in a recent review article [3], there is a lack of consensus about numerous issues related to PPCS including causation. However, considering predisposing, precipitating, and perpetuating factors appears to be a fruitful approach [4]. Nevertheless, PPCS are problematic because they decrease quality of life. For example, individuals with PPCS have reduced social interactions, difficulty continuing previously enjoyed past-times, and struggle resuming pre-injury physical capabilities, employment, and daily tasks [5]. Driving can also be impacted, with one study reporting that 93% of individuals with PPCS experience at least one difficulty that negatively impacted their driving [6].

Driving requires the integration of motor, cognitive, perceptual, and sensory skills in response to environmental information [7]. Sustaining a concussion may impact these driving abilities and result in impaired driving performance [6, 8, 9]. Furthermore, individuals who experienced a concussion but are no longer symptomatic exhibit impaired driving performance when assessed in a driving simulator [10]. Such impairments are also evident in on-road driving, where the number of motor vehicle collisions for persons six to nine years following a traumatic brain injury are more than double the reported average [11]. Accordingly, treatments are necessary to reduce the risk while driving following a concussion.

There are several challenges to treating individuals with PPCS. Individualized treatment plans that target physical and psychosocial symptoms are recommended [1, 12]. However, treatments focused on symptoms do not necessarily address their root cause, which may be altered brain physiology. Biofeedback approaches are designed to address physiological injury and may improve functional performance [13].

Heart rate variability (HRV) describes the natural beat-to-beat variability in heart rate. It represents autonomic function and sympathetic-parasympathetic balance [14]. HRV is altered in individuals suffering concussions [15] and PPCS, including hyperactive sympathetic activity and reduced parasympathetic activity [16]. HRV biofeedback is designed to repair sympathetic-parasympathetic balance, as well as baroreflex activity [17]. It improves cognitive functioning and emotional regulation in some individuals experiencing a brain injury [18]. It may also contribute to improved attention [19] and problem-solving abilities [20], and enhanced executive functioning [21]. HRV biofeedback may also reduce symptoms and improve mood in individuals with PPCS [22, 23].

HRV biofeedback is often used in conjunction with electroencephalograph (EEG) biofeedback (neurofeedback) since neurofeedback can also influence the neuroanatomical networks and structures that affect HRV [13, 24, 25]. Neurofeedback has evolved from measuring and training brain activity using surface electrodes, to more robust methods including source localization neurofeedback. This form of neurofeedback is known as low-resolution electromagnetic tomography (LoRETA) neurofeedback [26]. LoRETA neurofeedback allows the participant to see the amplitude of electrical activity at specific brain regions in real time, and they can therefore self-regulate this electrical activity [26]. It is non-invasive and enables individualized rehabilitation. Individualization is important as it is one of the biggest limitations of traditional brain injury interventions [12].

LoRETA neurofeedback corrects functional deficiencies in individuals with major depressive disorder [27]. When combined with HRV biofeedback, the intervention improves both depression and anxiety symptoms [28], which may contribute to improved driving performance and reduced driving errors [29, 30]. Additionally, the combined intervention may help individuals perceive, attend, and interpret a stimulus [7] by improving disorders of attentional processing [31, 32]. Following the interpretation of a stimulus, the driver must plan an action to react to a stimulus, and then execute the action [7]. LoRETA neurofeedback and HRV biofeedback may improve planning by improving executive function [32], and may improve execution by increasing motor [33] and impulse control [31]. Planning an action can also be improved through previous experience [7], and this may be improved through LoRETA neurofeedback and HRV biofeedback by way of improving working memory [34].

Therefore, this chapter describes a research study designed to determine whether HRV biofeedback in combination with LoRETA neurofeedback showed promise as an intervention to reduce self-reported concussive symptoms and improve simulated driving performance in individuals experiencing PPCS.

2. Materials and methods

Thirty-one individuals were recruited to participate in this study, which was approved by the Western University Health Science Research Ethics Board and registered with ClinicalTrials.gov (NCT03338036). Participants with PPCS had to be 18 years of age or older, experienced a clinically diagnosed concussion and completed a concussion rehabilitation program, and still experiencing ongoing symptoms. They also had to be fluent in English, hold a valid driver's license, and capable of using hand-held devices. Healthy participants had to be 18 years of age or older, and could not have experienced a concussion in the last two years. They also had to be fluent in English and hold a valid driver's license. All participants provided written informed consent.

Twenty-three individuals with PPCS were randomized into the intervention or active control group (11 in the intervention group and 12 in the PPCS control group). However, seven PPCS participants experienced a worsening of symptoms during the baseline testing and could not complete the driving simulator task, excluding them from participation. This resulted in seven participants in the intervention group (48.6 ± 14 years old, four females). The youngest participant in the intervention group was 30, while the oldest was 75. The PPCS control group had nine participants (54.7 ± 8 years old, six females), with the youngest being 37 and the oldest being 65. Lastly, there were eight healthy control participants (49.6 ± 16.5 years old, four females). The youngest healthy control participant was 25 while the oldest was 74.

2.1 Baseline and follow-up assessment

Participants were initially contacted via email about this study; their response prompted an informational email. They then met with a study investigator at the iMobile Research Lab at Western University, London, Ontario, Canada, where together they reviewed the letter of information. Once all questions were answered and they signed the consent form, the baseline assessment began.

The participant was first measured and fitted with a 19-lead EEG cap (Electro Cap International, Eaton, Ohio). Each electrode placement corresponded to specific locations on the scalp according to the 10–20 International System for electrode placement [35]. The electrodes were then filled with a water-soluble conducting gel (Electro-Gel, Electro Cap International, Eaton, Ohio). An abrasive gel (NuPrep) was used as skin preparation prior to attaching electrodes to both earlobes using clip electrodes; these sites acted as a reference. All leads used AFz as ground and passed through an amplifier (Evoke Neurosciences, New York, NY). Additionally, one electrode was taped to the participants chest, inferior to the left clavicle, to monitor their electrocardiogram.

The participant then completed a brain function assessment, including a three-minute resting EEG measurement with their eyes-closed. Afterwards, the participant completed a Rivermead Post-Concussion Symptoms Questionnaire

(RPQ) [36] and Generalized Anxiety Disorder 7-Item Scale (GAD-7) [37]. Next, they performed the driving simulation task on a CDS-200 DriveSafety™ simulator, which included a steering wheel and dash display from a Ford Focus, a gas and brake pedal, and three computer screens for displaying the environment around the vehicle. The simulator was adjusted for the participant's comfort, ensuring that they were the appropriate distance from the screens, and they were comfortable with the height and tilt of the steering wheel and distance to the pedals.

The simulation task began with a simulator acclimation protocol including dimmed lights to reduce visual strain, temperature control in the simulator room (21° C) to ensure comfort, utilization of a fan to increase air flow around the participant, and three acclimation drives totaling seven minutes. These factors have been identified to mitigate simulator sickness [38]. The acclimation drives increased in complexity, starting with a straight drive while maintaining a speed of approximately 50 kph with no other vehicles on the road and low visual complexity of the scenario. The next acclimation drive required navigating a city block with four consecutive left-hand turns, and ended with a drive requiring four consecutive right-hand turns. The left-hand and right-hand turn scenarios were completed with few vehicles on the road, thus introducing real driving situations. For example, the participant had to wait for an oncoming car to drive through the intersection before completing a left-hand turn. Participants were offered breaks between simulator tasks as needed. They were also screened for symptoms of simulator sickness before and after each acclimation drive using the Adapted Motion Sickness Assessment Questionnaire [39], adapted to an 11-point scale as done in previous research [40]. Participants rated their feelings of sweatiness, queasiness, dizziness, and nausea on a scale from 0 (not at all) to 10 (severely).

Finally, participants performed one of two simulator drives. Both drives contained the same scripted events representing potentially hazardous situations: an unexpected pedestrian crossing the street in front of the car, and a car suddenly pulling out of a driveway in front of the participant. The scripted events were pseudorandomized across the two drives to control for any potential learning effect of the route. The drive was approximately 10 minutes in length. These drives have been used in other experiments, and were specifically designed to assess the driving performance of young adults [40, 41].

After eight weeks, all participants returned to complete another brain function assessment, RPQ and GAD-7, and driving simulator acclimation and drive. The final simulator drive was the alternate drive to their baseline assessment. For example, if they completed Drive 1 in their baseline assessment, then they completed Drive 2 in their follow-up assessment.

2.2 Intervention

Participants in the intervention group received an Android tablet (either a Craig 7 inch 1 GB 6.0 "Marshmallow" Tablet, New York, New York or a Samsung Galaxy Tab A 7 inch 8 GB Android 5.1 "Lillipop" Tablet, Seoul, South Korea) and heart rate variability training tool (Evoke Waveband, Evoke Neurosciences, New York, New York) upon completion of their initial assessment. Participants in the intervention group were taught how to use the equipment, and instructed to perform a HRV biofeedback session every morning and night for eight weeks. Each HRV biofeedback session involved placing the Waveband just below their elbow, opening the application (Mindja, Evoke Neurosciences, New York, New York) on their tablet, and doing a 5-minute exercise in which they were cued to breathe at their resonant frequency [42]. Points were awarded as their HRV improved. Participants were also provided with a log book to record the dates and times of their completed sessions.

LoRETA neurofeedback sessions were performed in a private room at Parkwood Institute in London, Ontario. Each LoRETA neurofeedback session was broken up into 10 exposures, each two-minutes in duration, for a total of 20 minutes of training. Participants were instructed to "relax, focus, and turn on the green light", which would appear on a computer screen in front of them. The light turned green when the participants were appropriately activating the target cerebral areas at the appropriate amplitude, as determined from their initial assessment. Each participant in the intervention group was scheduled to participate in three sessions per week (usually at the same time on Mondays, Wednesdays, and Fridays), for eight consecutive weeks. This resulted in a potential total of 24 LoRETA neurofeedback sessions and 112 HRV biofeedback sessions.

2.3 Data analysis

Total scores on the GAD-7 for each participant were summed, and the change from baseline to follow-up was calculated. These changes were compared between the intervention, PPCS control, and healthy control groups using a Kruskal-Wallis non-parametric analysis (SPSS 25, IBM Corp., Armonk, NY). RPQ outcomes were tallied as two scores, similarly to previous research [43]. The headache, nausea and dizziness scores were tallied together (RPQ-3), and the remaining questions were tallied separately (RPQ-13). The differences from baseline to follow-up between the three participant groups in both RPQ sub scores were also assessed using a Kruskal-Wallis analysis.

Driving simulation analysis focused on two scripted events (an unexpected pedestrian crossing and a car suddenly pulling out of a driveway), as these events challenged the participant's reactions. Three parameters were assessed for these events: reaction time, maximum brake applied and the distance from the event when the maximum brake was applied. Reaction times were quantified as the time difference between the start of the hazardous event and when the participant applied pressure to the brake or suddenly changed their lane deviation (i.e. swerving). Maximum brake applied was indicated on a zero to one scale, with zero representing no braking and one representing the maximum brake application possible. Differences from baseline to follow-up between the three participant groups were analyzed using a non-parametric Kruskal-Wallis analysis.

3. Results

3.1 Compliance

Participants in the intervention group attended 88% of their LoRETA neurofeedback sessions (21 ± 2.6 of the 24 possible sessions; the 25, 50, and 75th percentiles were 18.5, 22 and 23, respectively). The range extended from a low of 17 (one participant) to a maximum of 24 (two participants). Additionally, participants on average completed 86% of their HRV sessions (96.7 ± 10.1 of the 112 possible sessions; the 25, 50, and 75th percentiles were 86, 99, and 106, respectively). The range extended from a low of 83 (two participants) to a maximum of 111 (one participant).

3.2 GAD-7 and RPQ

There were no significant differences in GAD-7 or RPQ-13 between the intervention, PPCS control, and healthy control groups (**Table 1**). There were significant differences in RPQ-3 outcomes. Post-hoc analysis revealed significant differences between the intervention group and healthy control group ($p < .05$) and the PPCS control and healthy control groups ($p < .05$). The difference between the intervention and PPCS control group was not significant ($p = .83$). Furthermore, participants demonstrated variable responses, therefore individual measures are presented for GAD-7 (**Figure 1**), RPQ-3 (**Figure 2**), and RPQ-13 (**Figure 3**).

Outcome	Intervention	PPCS Control	Healthy Control	*H* Statistic	*p* Value
GAD-7 (Median)	−2.3	−0.6	−1.5	0.94	.62
RPQ-3 (Median)	−1	−3	5.5	12.02	<.01*
RPQ-13 (Mean rank)	13.2	13.0	16.2	0.88	.65
Car pull out reaction time (Mean rank)	7.7	13.0	9.7	2.88	.24
Car pull out max brake (0–1; Median)	−.14	0.00	−.05	0.97	.62
Car pull out distance at brake max (m; Median)	2.47	−2.70	−0.65	3.66	.16
Pedestrian walk out reaction time (s; Median)	−0.48	0.53	−0.08	1.19	.55
Pedestrian walk out max brake (0–1; Median)	0.00	−.03	−.03	0.02	.99
Pedestrian walk out distance at brake max (Mean rank)	12.3	10.0	9.1	1.05	.59

Table 1.
*Statistical evaluations of the change in generalized anxiety disorder 7-item scale (GAD-7), Rivermead post-concussion symptoms questionnaire (RPQ), and driving outcomes from baseline to follow-up. *indicates statistical significance.*

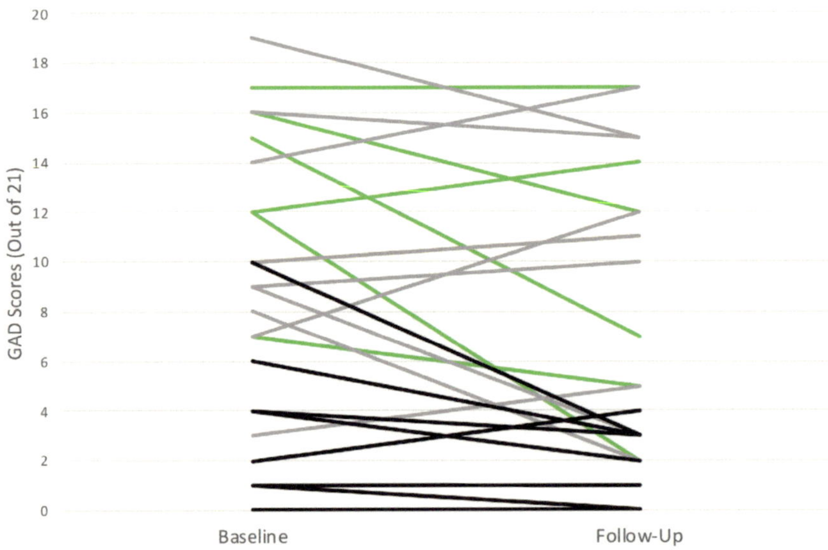

Figure 1.
GAD-7 scores for individual participants. Green indicates participants in the intervention group, gray indicates PPCS controls, and black indicates healthy controls.

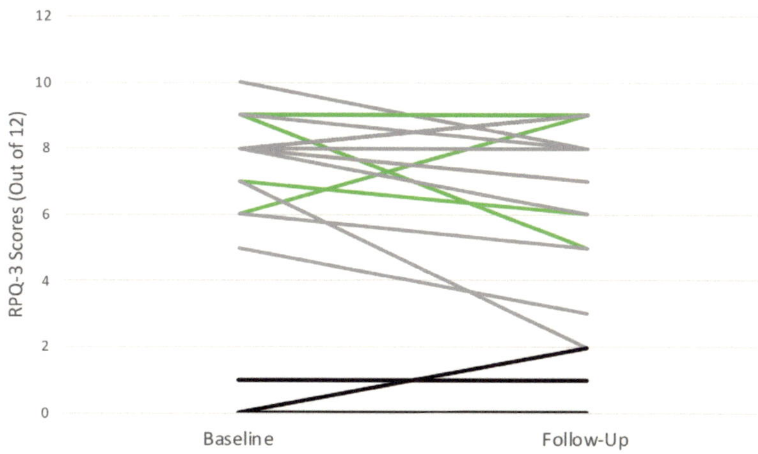

Figure 2.
RPQ-3 scores for individual participants. Green indicates participants in the intervention group, gray indicates PPCS controls, and black indicates healthy controls.

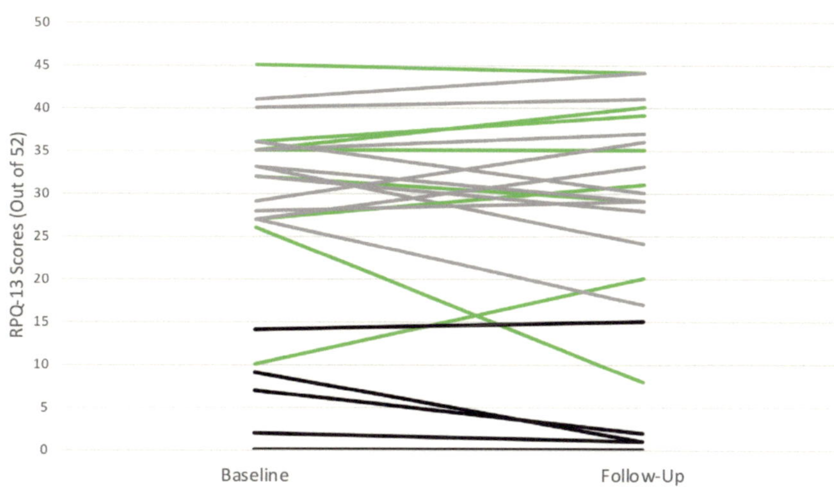

Figure 3.
RPQ-13 scores for individual participants. Green indicates participants in the intervention group, gray indicates PPCS controls, and black indicates healthy controls.

3.3 Driving simulation

Ten participants were involved in a collision during their driving simulator performances. Eight collisions occurred in the baseline assessment (two from the intervention group, two from the PPCS control group, and four from the healthy control group) and two occurred in their follow-up assessment (both from the PPCS control group). Collisions automatically terminated the simulation. Two collisions occurred after the scripted events. Accordingly, full drive metrics were not available for eight participants. The analysis of changes in reaction time to the car suddenly pulling out of the driveway were based on seven intervention participants, six PPCS control participants, and six healthy controls. There were no differences between groups in reaction time to the car suddenly pulling out, or their maximum brake effort or distance (**Table 1**).

Collisions also effectively reduced the number of participants that were exposed to the unexpected pedestrian crossing. The change in reaction time in response to the unexpected pedestrian crossing was based on six intervention participants, seven PPCS control participants, and eight healthy controls. There were no differences between groups in their reaction time, maximum brake effort or distance to an unexpected pedestrian crossing (**Table 1**).

4. Discussion

Our intervention evaluated a combination of LoRETA neurofeedback and HRV biofeedback in individuals with PPCS, and compared concussive symptoms and driving performance to participants with PPCS that did not receive the intervention, and a healthy control group. Individuals in the intervention group reported improvements in RPQ-3 outcomes compared to the healthy control group. However, the PPCS control group also had reduced RPQ-3 outcomes compared to the healthy control group, and the difference between the intervention and PPCS control group was not significant. There were no statistically significant differences in GAD-7 scores or driving simulation outcomes (reaction time, maximum brake or distance at maximum brake) to the scripted events of the car suddenly pulling out of a driveway or the unexpected pedestrian crossing. Therefore, the results of this study indicate that LoRETA neurofeedback and HRV biofeedback did not reduce symptom number or severity, nor did it improve simulated driving performance. However, outcomes varied between participants. Emerging models evaluating the predisposing, precipitating, and perpetuating factors related to PPCS [4] may provide insights into the variable responses between participants, and should be considered in future investigations.

Previous research has shown that a single session of LoRETA neurofeedback results in acute changes in current densities in specific regions of the brain [27]. As well, previous intervention studies have indicated that LoRETA neurofeedback reduced symptoms in individuals with a brain injury [44, 45]. But, these studies tailored the LoRETA neurofeedback protocol for each individual. Furthermore, the target cerebral areas and training amplitudes also varied between studies based on the individual initial assessments. Despite our utilization of an initial EEG assessment, other factors could have been considered to inform cerebral area and amplitude selection, and further individualize our protocol.

Previous research has recommended considering initial symptom presentation when creating a LoRETA neurofeedback protocol to treat acute brain injuries [46]. Initial symptom presentation was difficult to attain in our study because participants were no longer in the acute phase of their injury. Therefore, this increased the risk of recall bias because of this population's increased likelihood for impaired memory recall [47]. However, it is unclear whether considering initial symptom presentation, current symptom presentation, or a combination may be more appropriate when creating a LoRETA neurofeedback protocol for individuals with PPCS. Secondly, the number of sessions should be based on the rate of improvement rather than a fixed number of sessions [46], which we chose to maintain for a consistent research protocol. The 24-session protocol was recommended by a licensed practitioner to balance intervention effects, research feasibility, and participant compliance. Lastly, consideration of persisting symptoms and their severity may further refine the intervention to increase participant's improvements. For example, there is a hyperbolic relationship between initial symptom presentation and number of neurofeedback sessions necessary [46], with increased initial symptoms requiring more neurofeedback sessions. Similarly, an increase in symptom persistence could increase the number of neurofeedback sessions required for improvement. Consideration of these three factors may have influenced the participants' responses to the intervention.

The lack of improvement in the driving simulation may have also been a result of the complex relationship between the outcome measures in this study. Outcomes (symptoms and driving simulation metrics) were evaluated independently, but there may not be a direct relationship between symptoms and driving simulation performance. Other studies have used structural equation modeling to evaluate similar types of relationships [48], but this was not possible in the current experiment due to the limited number of participants.

Individuals with a concussion or PPCS often experience executive dysfunction [47], which may be exhibited by inappropriate driving speed, following others too closely, or braking at inappropriate times [49]. Participants in the intervention group exhibited the greatest decreases in reaction times to the hazardous events (pedestrian walking out and car pulling out). Although these changes were not statistically significant, improved reaction times may indicate improved processing times, which is associated with fewer collisions [50]. Additionally, participants in the intervention group had the largest increases in distance from the hazardous event when they maximally applied the brake. They also exhibited the largest decrease in maximum brake effort when the car pulled out (although not statistically significant). These improvements also indicate increased driving safety, as increased distance and decreased brake effort indicate improved decision-making and ultimately improved executive function [49]. These safety improvements are particularly important for the PPCS population as their risk of collision may be higher when compared to the normal population [51].

The results of this study further indicate that individuals with PPCS require specialized driving evaluations, as previously identified [6, 9, 52, 53]. However, only half of physicians 'almost always' provide driving guidance following a concussion [54]. The lack of universally accepted procedures may be related to the absence of return-to-drive guidelines. Current clinical practice guidelines suggest that individuals who experience a concussion should not drive for 24 hours post-injury [55]. However, there are no guidelines for individuals driving with persistent symptoms, nor graded return to driving. This absence of clinical guidelines to assist physicians in making fitness to drive determinations in this population may increase the risk of collisions in individuals with PPCS. Additionally, 30% of physicians have stated that they do not have clear 'return-to-drive criteria' when evaluating fitness to drive in recently concussed individuals [54]. This further illustrates the need for research on the driving performance of individuals with PPCS, which can inform evidence-based return-to-drive guidelines. As indicated by this study, driving simulation research in this population is limited by the likelihood of simulator sickness, as occurred with seven of our recruited participants. This represents a barrier for completing this type of research. However, simulator sickness mitigation protocols can help reduce the incidence and improve retention.

Our study has shown some promising results, but does have some limitations. Most importantly, this study examined the effects of neurofeedback and HRV biofeedback on a small sample size. This represents a challenge with respect to both internal validity and generalizability [56]. For instance, our sample of participants may be biased towards high-functioning individuals that did not experience simulator sickness. Our study also did not consider medication usage that may have influenced participants' outcome scores [1]. Another potential limitation was that we did not consider driving experience. Although there were no significant differences between age groups, some individuals may have had more experience driving or more driving training. This could have resulted in differences in driving simulation performance prior to a brain injury. Additionally, although our parameterization of the RPQ is similar to previous research [43], other research indicates the RPQ can be quantified using a four factor model, clustered as vision, vertigo, mood/

somatic and cognitive domains [57]. It is unclear how our parameterization of the RPQ scores may have influenced the findings. Lastly, this study only looked at the immediate effects of the LoRETA neurofeedback and HRV biofeedback intervention. Although consistent with other neurofeedback studies [31, 58, 59], it is unclear whether short-term responses reflect long-term outcomes. Alternatively, there may be delays before symptoms change [1], and accordingly a reduction in symptoms could also be delayed.

This study is the first to systematically implement and evaluate the outcomes of a LORETA neurofeedback and HRV biofeedback protocol for civilians with PPCS. It is also noteworthy that this study evaluated the outcomes of LORETA neurofeedback and HRV biofeedback in individuals that completed a rehabilitation program and had ongoing PPCS; a population with symptoms that may be difficult to treat [47]. Considering the participant population, these results are especially valuable to healthcare practitioners because they include clinically relevant outcomes (i.e. self-reported symptoms and driving performance).

5. Conclusions

This study implemented an intervention involving a combination of LoRETA neurofeedback and HRV biofeedback for eight weeks, based on individual EEG baseline assessments. Eleven participants with PPCS were included in the intervention group (seven that finished the protocol), 12 in the PPCS control group (nine that finished the protocol), and eight healthy control participants. Considering the PPCS intervention group as a whole, this combined intervention did not improve symptoms or driving simulation performance. However, some of the individuals did show improvements. This may indicate that this intervention is effective for a subgroup of individuals with PPCS, or perhaps that the intervention needs to be further individualized to optimize participants' responses. Specifically, the nature of the symptoms, rate of improvement, and length of symptom persistence may need to be considered to individualize the protocol. The results of this study also emphasize the importance of evaluating fitness to drive following a concussion, as well as the need for return-to-drive guidelines for individuals experiencing symptoms following a concussion.

Acknowledgements

We would like to thank Shannon McGuire, Dalton Wolfe, and the staff of the Acquired Brain Injury Outpatient program at Parkwood Institute for donating research space and helping to recruit participants.

Conflict of interest

Dr. James Thompson is the Co-Founder of Evoke Neuroscience. Evoke Neuroscience donated the eVox EEG systems for this research, and the corresponding analyses. Dr. Thompson contributed to the research design, analysis and manuscript editing. All remaining authors have no conflict of interest to report.

Author details

Marquise M. Bonn[1], Liliana Alvarez[1], James W.G. Thompson[2] and James P. Dickey[1*]

1 Faculty of Health Sciences, Western University, London, Canada

2 Evoke Neuroscience Inc., New York, USA

*Address all correspondence to: jdickey@uwo.ca

References

[1] McCrory P, Meeuwisse W, Dvorak J, Aubry M, Bailes J, Broglio S, et al. Consensus statement on concussion in sport-the 5th international conference on concussion in sport held in Berlin, October 2016. British Journal of Sports Medicine. 2018;**51**(11):838-847

[2] Voormolen DC, Cnossen MC, Polinder S, von Steinbuechel N, Vos PE, Haagsma JA. Divergent classification methods of post-concussion syndrome after mild traumatic brain injury: Prevalence rates, risk factors, and functional outcome. Journal of Neurotrauma. 2018;**35**(11):1233-1241

[3] Young G. Thirty complexities and controversies in mild traumatic brain injury and persistent post-concussion syndrome: a roadmap for research and practice. Psychological Injury and Law. 2020;**13**:427-451

[4] Rickards TA, Cranston CC, McWhorter J. Persistent post-concussive symptoms: A model of predisposing, precipitating, and perpetuating factors. Applied Neuropsychology: Adult.;2020; In press:1-111

[5] Emanuelson I, Andersson Holmkvist E, Björklund R, Stålhammar D. Quality of life and post-concussion symptoms in adults after mild traumatic brain injury: A population-based study in western Sweden. Acta Neurologica Scandinavica. 2003;**108**(5):332-338

[6] Bottari C, Lamothe M-P, Gosselin N, Gélinas I, Ptito A. Driving difficulties and adaptive strategies: the perception of individuals having sustained a mild traumatic brain injury. Rehabilitation Research and Practice. 2012;**2012**: Article ID 837301.

[7] Rizzo M, Kellison IL. The brain on the road. In: Marcotte TD, Grant I, editors. Neuropsychology of Everyday Functioning. New York, NY, US: Guilford Press; 2010. pp. 168-208

[8] Dumphy D, Zerpa C, Hoshizaki T, Weaver B, McKee D, Bédard M, et al. The effect of concussion on reaction time and dual tasking ability in a simulated driving environment. ISBS Proceedings Archive. 2017;**35**(1):166

[9] Preece MH, Horswill MS, Geffen GM. Driving after concussion: The acute effect of mild traumatic brain injury on drivers' hazard perception. Neuropsychology. 2010;**24**(4):493

[10] Schmidt JD, Hoffman NL, Ranchet M, Miller LS, Tomporowski PD, Akinwuntan AE, et al. Driving after concussion: Is it safe to drive after symptoms resolve? Journal of Neurotrauma. 2017;**34**(8):1571-1578

[11] Schanke A, Rike P, Mølmen A, Østen P. Driving behaviour after brain injury: A follow-up of accident rate and driving patterns 6-9 years post-injury. Journal of Rehabilitation Medicine. 2008;**40**(9):733-736

[12] Rees L, Marshall S, Hartridge C, Mackie D, Weiser M, Erabi G. Cognitive interventions post acquired brain injury. Brain Injury. 2007;**21**(2):161-200

[13] Thompson M, Thompson L, Reid-Chung A. Treating Postconcussion syndrome with LORETA z-score neurofeedback and heart rate variability biofeedback: Neuroanatomical/neurophysiological rationale, methods, and case examples. Biofeedback. 2015;**43**(1):15-26

[14] Pomeranz B, Macaulay RJ, Caudill MA, Kutz I, Adam D, Gordon D, et al. Assessment of autonomic function in humans by heart rate spectral analysis. American Journal of Physiology: Heart and Circulatory Physiology. 1985;**248**(1):H151-H153

[15] Thompson J, Hagedorn D. Multimodal analysis: New approaches to the concussion conundrum. Journal of Clinical Sport Psychology. 2012;**6**(1):22-46

[16] Gall B, Parkhouse W, Goodman D. Heart rate variability of recently concussed athletes at rest and exercise. Medicine and Science in Sports and Exercise. 2004;**36**:1269-1274

[17] Lehrer PM, Vaschillo E, Vaschillo B, Lu S-E, Eckberg DL, Edelberg R, et al. Heart rate variability biofeedback increases baroreflex gain and peak expiratory flow. Psychosomatic Medicine. 2003;**65**(5):796-805

[18] Francis HM, Fisher A, Rushby JA, McDonald S. Reduced heart rate variability in chronic severe traumatic brain injury: Association with impaired emotional and social functioning, and potential for treatment using biofeedback. Neuropsychological Rehabilitation. 2016;**26**(1):103-125

[19] Hansen AL, Johnsen BH, Thayer JF. Vagal influence on working memory and attention. International Journal of Psychophysiology. 2003;**48**(3):263-274

[20] Kim S, Zemon V, Cavallo MM, Rath JF, McCraty R, Foley FW. Heart rate variability biofeedback, executive functioning and chronic brain injury. Brain Injury. 2013;**27**(2):209-222

[21] Hansen AL, Johnsen BH, Sollers JJ 3rd, Stenvik K, Thayer JF. Heart rate variability and its relation to prefrontal cognitive function: The effects of training and detraining. European Journal of Applied Physiology. 2004;**93**(3):263-272

[22] Lagos L, Thompson J, Vaschillo E. A preliminary study: Heart rate variability biofeedback for treatment of Postconcussion syndrome. Biofeedback. 2013;**41**(3):136-143

[23] Kim S, Rath JF, McCraty R, Zemon V, Cavallo MM, Foley FW. Heart rate variability biofeedback, self-regulation, and severe brain injury. Biofeedback. 2015;**43**(1):6-14

[24] Bhandari T, Thompson L, Reid-Chung A. Treating postconcussion syndrome using neurofeedback: A case study. Biofeedback. 2013;**41**(4):174-182

[25] Shaw L, Zaichkowsky L, Wilson V. Setting the balance: Using biofeedback and neurofeedback with gymnasts. Journal of Clinical Sport Psychology. 2012;**6**(1):47-66

[26] Congedo M, Lubar JF, Joffe D. Low-resolution electromagnetic tomography neurofeedback. IEEE Transactions on Neural Systems and Rehabilitation Engineering. 2004;**12**(4):387-397

[27] Zotev V, Bodurka J. Effects of simultaneous real-time fMRI and EEG neurofeedback in major depressive disorder evaluated with brain electromagnetic tomography. Neuroimage: Clinical. 2020 2020;**28**: 102459

[28] White EK, Groeneveld KM, Tittle RK, Bolhuis NA, Martin RE, Royer TG, et al. Combined neurofeedback and heart rate variability training for individuals with symptoms of anxiety and depression: A retrospective study. NeuroRegulation. 2017;**4**(1):37-55

[29] Bulmash EL, Moller HJ, Kayumov L, Shen J, Wang X, Shapiro CM. Psychomotor disturbance in depression: Assessment using a driving simulator paradigm. Journal of Affective Disorders. 2006;**93**(1-3):213-218

[30] Wong IY, Mahar D, Titchener K. Driven by distraction: Investigating the effects of anxiety on driving performance using the attentional control theory. Journal of Risk Research. 2015;**18**(10):1293-1306

[31] Kaiser DA, Othmer S. Effect of neurofeedback on variables of attention in a large multi-center trial. Journal of Neurotherapy. 2000;**4**(1):5-15

[32] Wigton NL, Krigbaum G. Attention, executive function, behavior, and electrocortical function, significantly improved with 19-channel z-score neurofeedback in a clinical setting: A pilot study. Journal of Attention Disorders. 2019;**23**(4):398-408

[33] Wing K. Effect of neurofeedback on motor recovery of a patient with brain injury: A case study and its implications for stroke rehabilitation. Topics in Stroke Rehabilitation. 2001;**8**(3):45-53

[34] Keizer AW, Verment RS, Hommel B. Enhancing cognitive control through neurofeedback: A role of gamma-band activity in managing episodic retrieval. NeuroImage. 2010;**49**(4):3404-3413

[35] Jasper HH. The ten-twenty electrode system of the international federation. Electroencephalography and Clinical Neurophysiology. 1958;**10**:371-375

[36] King NS, Crawford S, Wenden FJ, Moss NEG, Wade DT. The Rivermead post concussion symptoms questionnaire: A measure of symptoms commonly experienced after head injury and its reliability. Journal of Neurology. 1995;**242**(9):587-592

[37] Spitzer RL, Kroenke K, Williams JB, Lowe B. A brief measure for assessing generalized anxiety disorder: The GAD-7. Archives of Internal Medicine. 2006;**166**(10):1092-1097

[38] Classen S, Bewernitz M, Shechtman O. Driving simulator sickness: An evidence-based review of the literature. American Journal of Occupational Therapy. 2011;**65**(2):179-188

[39] Gianaros PJ, Muth ER, Mordkoff JT, Levine ME, Stern RM. A questionnaire for the assessment of the multiple dimensions of motion sickness. Aviation Space and Environmental Medicine. 2001;**72**(2):115-119

[40] Alvarez L, Classen S, Medhizadah S, Knott M, He W. Pilot efficacy of a DriveFocus intervention on the driving performance of young drivers. Frontiers in Public Health. 2018;**6**:125

[41] Alvarez L, Classen S, Medhizadah S, Knott M, Asantey K, He W, et al. Feasibility of DriveFocus and driving simulation interventions in Young drivers. OTJR: Occupation, Participation and Health. 2018;**38**(4):245-253

[42] Lehrer PM, Vaschillo E, Vaschillo B. Resonant frequency biofeedback training to increase cardiac variability: Rationale and manual for training. Applied Psychophysiology and Biofeedback. 2000;**25**(3):177-191

[43] Eyres S, Carey A, Gilworth G, Neumann V, Tennant A. Construct validity and reliability of the Rivermead post-concussion symptoms questionnaire. Clinical Rehabilitation. 2005;**19**(8):878-887

[44] Nelson DV, Esty ML. Neurotherapy for chronic headache following traumatic brain injury. Military Medical Research. 2015;**2**:22

[45] Surmeli T, Eralp E, Mustafazade I, KosIH,OzerGE,SurmeliOH.Quantitative EEG Neurometric analysis-guided neurofeedback treatment in Postconcussion syndrome (PCS): Forty cases. How is Neurometric analysis important for the treatment of PCS and as a biomarker? Clinical EEG and Neuroscience. 2017;48(3): 217-230.

[46] Bounias M, Laibow RE, Stubblebine AN, Sandground H, Bonaly A. EEG-NeuroBioFeedback treatment of patients with brain injury part 4: Duration of treatments

as a function of both the initial load of clinical symptoms and the rate of rehabilitation. Journal of Neurotherapy. 2002;**6**(1):23-38

[47] Ontario Neurotrauma Foundation. Guidelines for concussion/mild traumatic brain injury & persistent symptoms: for adults (18+ years of age): Ontario Neurotrauma Foundation; 2018.

[48] Ullman JB. Bentler PM. Structural equation modeling. Handbook of Psychology. Second Edition; 2012

[49] Kraft M, Amick MM, Barth JT, French LM, Lew HL. A review of driving simulator parameters relevant to the operation enduring freedom/operation Iraqi freedom veteran population. American Journal of Physical Medicine and Rehabilitation. 2010;**89**(4):336-344

[50] Fergenson PE. The relationship between information processing and driving accident and violation record. Human Factors. 2016;**13**(2):173-176

[51] Bernstein JPK, Calamia M. Assessing the longer-term effects of mild traumatic brain injury on self-reported driving ability. Physical Medicine & Rehabilitation. 2018;**10**(11):1153-1163

[52] Lane AK, Benoit D. Driving, brain injury and assistive technology. NeuroRehabilitation. 2011;**28**(3):221-229

[53] Lindsay S, Stoica A. A systematic review of factors affecting driving and public transportation among youth and young adults with acquired brain injury. Brain Injury. 2017;**31**(10):1257-1269

[54] Lucas JA, Moore JB, Davis S, Brooks JO, Miles C. Provider attitudes and management regarding returning to drive after concussion. British Journal of Sports Medicine. 2018;**53**(8):495

[55] Marshall S, Bayley M, McCullagh S, Velikonja D, Berrigan L, Ouchterlony D, et al. Updated clinical practice guidelines for concussion/mild traumatic brain injury and persistent symptoms. Brain Injury. 2015;**29**(6):688-700

[56] Shekelle PG, Morton SC, Suttorp MJ, Buscemi N, Friesen C. Agency for Healthcare R, et al. challenges in systematic reviews of complementary and alternative medicine topics. Annals of Internal Medicine. 2005;**142**(12 Pt 2):1042-1047

[57] Thomas M, Skilbeck C, Cannan P, Slatyer M. The structure of the Rivermead post-concussion symptoms questionnaire in Australian adults with traumatic brain injury. Brain Impairment. 2017;**19**(2):166-182

[58] Raymond J, Varney C, Parkinson LA, Gruzelier JH. The effects of alpha/theta neurofeedback on personality and mood. Cognitive Brain Research. 2005;**23**(2-3):287-292

[59] Gevensleben H, Holl B, Albrecht B, Vogel C, Schlamp D, Kratz O, et al. Is neurofeedback an efficacious treatment for ADHD? A randomised controlled clinical trial. Journal of Child Psychology and Psychiatry and Allied Disciplines. 2009;**50**(7):780-789

Chapter 4

The Influence of Sagittal Plane Spine Alignment on Neurophysiology and Sensorimotor Control Measures: Optimization of Function through Structural Correction

Paul A. Oakley, Ibrahim M. Moustafa and Deed E. Harrison

Abstract

Increasingly, there is more attention being directed to the role that full spine sagittal alignment plays in causing or exacerbating a variety of musculoskeletal disorders. Similarly, spinal displacements, termed subluxation, are thought to cause dysfunctions in the entire neuromusculoskeletal system that may lead to altered neurophysiological function, abnormal sensorimotor control, and altered autonomic nervous system function. Abnormalities in neutral upright spine alignment (sagittal translation or flexion deformities) are known to increase mechanical loads (stresses and strains) on the central nervous system. These increased mechanical loads may subtly or overtly impair neurophysiological function as measured with evoked potentials in terms of latency and amplitudes of potentials. Proprioceptive afferentation from spine ligaments, muscles and discs are considered a major component of sensorimotor control. The voluminous mechanoreceptors in spinal muscles, ligaments, and discs plays an intimate role, providing the necessary neurophysiological input in a feed forward and feedback system for sensorimotor control via connections to the vestibular, visual and central nervous systems. Of particular interest, a network of neurophysiological connections between spine mechanoreceptors and the sympathetic nervous system has been documented. This chapter explores the hypothesis and evidence that restoring normal posture and spine alignment has important influences on neurophysiology, sensorimotor control and autonomic nervous system functionality. There is limited but high-quality research identifying that sagittal spine alignment restoration plays an important role in improving neurophysiology, sensorimotor control, and autonomic nervous system function. Accordingly, in the current chapter, we review this work in hopes of stimulating further investigations into structural rehabilitation of the spine and posture.

Keywords: spinal deformity, sensorimotor control, sagittal plane alignment, sympathetic skin resistance, dermatomal somatosensory evoked potentials, spine rehabilitation

1. Introduction

A normal spine alignment including coronal and sagittal balance is essential for optimal biomechanical function [1–7]. The spine, which allows for simultaneous stability and mobility, also has the inherent role of housing and protecting the brain and spinal cord. The alignment of the spine is critical in the context of allowing normal function of the central nervous system (CNS); that is, by not impeding its function by various loading mechanisms (i.e. overstretching the nervous tissues) [8, 9]. Clinical trials [10–16] and case reports [17–25] have demonstrated that corrections in patient posture have resulted in relief of neurological symptoms including for example, cervical spondylotic and discogenic radiculopathy, cervical spondylotic myelopathy (CSM), lumbosacral discogenic radiculopathy, trigeminal neuralgia (TN), dystonia, Parkinson's disease (PD), carpal tunnel syndrome (CTS), and Tourette's syndrome (TS). Although the precise mechanisms underlying improved neurological function in patients having improved postural alignment are not fully understood, they are thought to lie in the biomechanics of the CNS and in normalization of load sharing across tissues innervated by mechanoreceptors which are integral in sensorimotor control through somatosensory potentials.

In 1960, a monograph was published by Alf Breig documenting for the first time, the most comprehensive illustrative demonstrations of the biomechanics of the central nervous system (CNS) [8]. This seminal work laid the groundwork for the comprehensive understanding of how spine movement affects the CNS; that is, how physiologic deformation of the cord and brainstem simultaneously accompanies normal postural movements of the spine (i.e. 'neurodynamics'). In 1978, Breig published a second book expanding on the concepts outlined in 1960, and focused on 'adverse mechanical tension' in the CNS and how this produces common neurological symptoms and signs [9]. An exciting development by Breig was his invention of the 'cervicolordodesis' surgical procedure that increased the cervical lordosis and prevented cervical flexion to relieve tension within the cord, brainstem and nerve roots demonstrating dramatic improvements of neurological disorders including nerve root compression syndromes, TN, multiple sclerosis (MS) and other neuromusculoskeletal conditions [26].

A second prevailing theory on how normalization of spine/posture alignment can dramatically alter patient pain, disability, function, and neurophysiology is through cervical spine sensory afferent input (so called afferentation) and its influence on the motor system termed sensorimotor control. As a result of activation of mechanoreceptors contained in the various ligaments, discs, muscles and skin, changes in spine position-alignment has a major influence on motor control [27]. Intimate connections exist between afferent input (from the proprioceptive, visual and vestibular systems) and stable upright postures of the head and neck [28]. The mechanoreceptors in the cervical spine soft tissues provide necessary neurophysiological input in a feed forward and feedback system for sensorimotor control via connections to the vestibular, visual and central nervous systems [29]. Furthermore, a complex network of neurophysiological connections between cervical spine mechanoreceptors and the sympathetic nervous system exists [30–32]. Though the effects of autonomic system activity on musculoskeletal function has been extensively studied, there is a paucity of research demonstrating that the autonomic nervous system is intimately responsive to changes in the afferent articular input due to spine joint dysfunction [33]. Alterations in afferent articular input driven by spine joint aberrant movement (altered kinematics) and subtle or overt tissue damage is generally referred to as 'dysafferentation' in the literature. The assumption that restoring normal posture and cervical spine alignment is important for a better afferentation process and improved autonomic nervous system function has some preliminary evidence in the recent literature [10, 34].

Today there are non-surgical evidence-based techniques known to improve posture and spine alignment; in essence to accomplish what Breig was able to do, only without surgery (e.g. increase cervical lordosis). One of these methods is Chiropractic BioPhysics® (CBP®) technique which is a full-spine and posture treatment that utilizes mirror image® (i.e. 'corrective') exercises, adjustments and spinal traction procedures to restore normal spine alignment [35–39]. Due to the implicit interconnectedness of spine alignment and neurologic function, these methods are proving to be particularly effective in treating patients with neurological and sensorimotor control disorders, where perhaps unknowingly, poor spine alignment is a causative factor in patients suffering from neurologic ailments in which their symptoms are exacerbated and/or directly caused by the adverse nerve tensions placed upon them and by dysafferentation caused by spine and postural deviations (i.e. adult spinal deformity/subluxation).

This chapter reviews the Harrison normal spinal model [40–47] that is used to assess a patient's spine alignment as compared to the normal/ideal position (i.e. gold standard), how the central nervous system is housed in and biomechanically functions within the skeletal structure under normal and pathologic conditions, including mechanisms for neurologic symptom generation under pathologic biomechanical tensions, and altered sensorimotor control from dysafferentation driven by altered load sharing and spine kinematics. Simultaneously, the CBP structural rehabilitation approach to realigning the spine and postural position in order to treat patients who present with spinal subluxation that is suspected to be pathognomonic for their pain, disability, and generalized neurologic sensorimotor disorders will be a main theme.

2. The Harrison normal spinal model

Any contemporary discussion about the normal/ideal human spinal configuration is regarding its precise orientation (i.e. precise shape of the different spinal regions). Although many research groups have attempted to model the shape of the normal human spine, few have done so as comprehensively and systematically as the Harrison group [40–47]. In a series of studies, elliptical shape modeling of the path of the posterior longitudinal ligament was performed on radiograph samples of asymptomatic subjects. Computer iterations of spine shape modeling was used to determine a best-fit geometric spinal shape by fitting various ellipses of altered minor-to-major axis ratios to the digitized posterior vertebral body corners of the cervical [40–42], thoracic [43, 44], and lumbar spinal regions [45–47] (**Figure 1**).

The Harrison normal spine model (**Figure 1**) features a circular cervical lordosis, and portions of an elliptical curve for both the thoracic kyphosis (more curvature cephalad), and lumbar lordosis (more curvature caudad). Consequently, features of the normal human spine reveal that the opposite thoracic and lumbar curves meet together at the thoraco-lumbar junction being essentially straight; the upper, deeper curve of the upper thoracic spine reflects oppositely at the cervico-thoracic junction (between T1 and T2) and continues into the cervical lordosis; the lower lumbar spine increases its lordotic alignment having two-thirds of its curve between L4-S1 as it meets the forward tilted sacral base. The spine is modeled as vertical in the front view. The spine alignment is easily quantified by repeatable and reliable methods from measuring its position from standing X-rays [48–52] (**Figure 2**).

The Harrison normal spine model has been validated in several ways. Simple analyses of alignment data of normal asymptomatic populations have been done [40–47, 53]. Comparison studies between normal samples to symptomatic samples [40, 41, 53]; as well as between normal samples to theoretical ideal models have

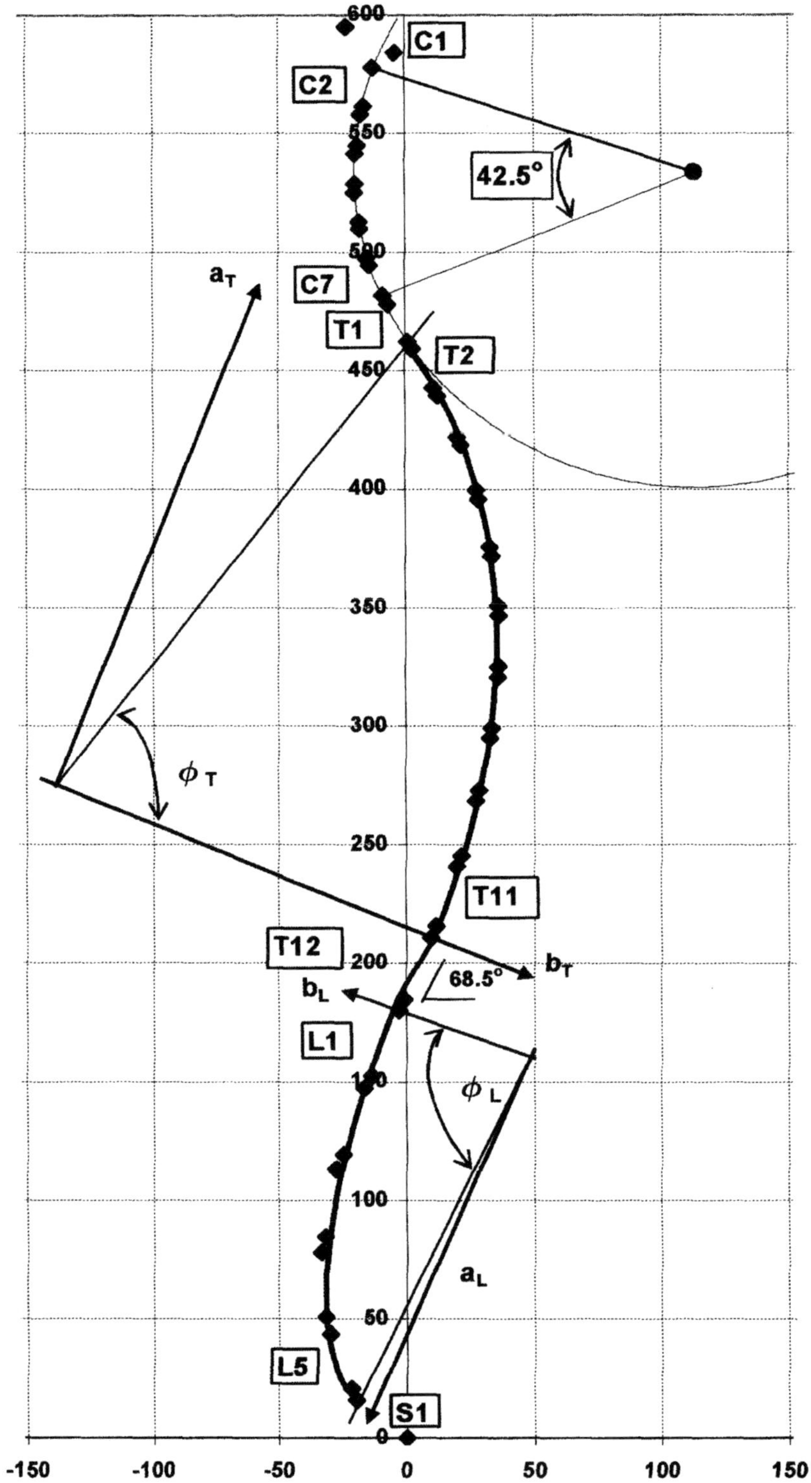

Figure 1.
The Harrison normal sagittal spine model as the path of the posterior longitudinal ligament. The cervical, thoracic and lumbar curves are all portions of an elliptical curve having a unique minor-to-major axis ratio. The cervical curve is circular meaning the minor and major axes are equal.

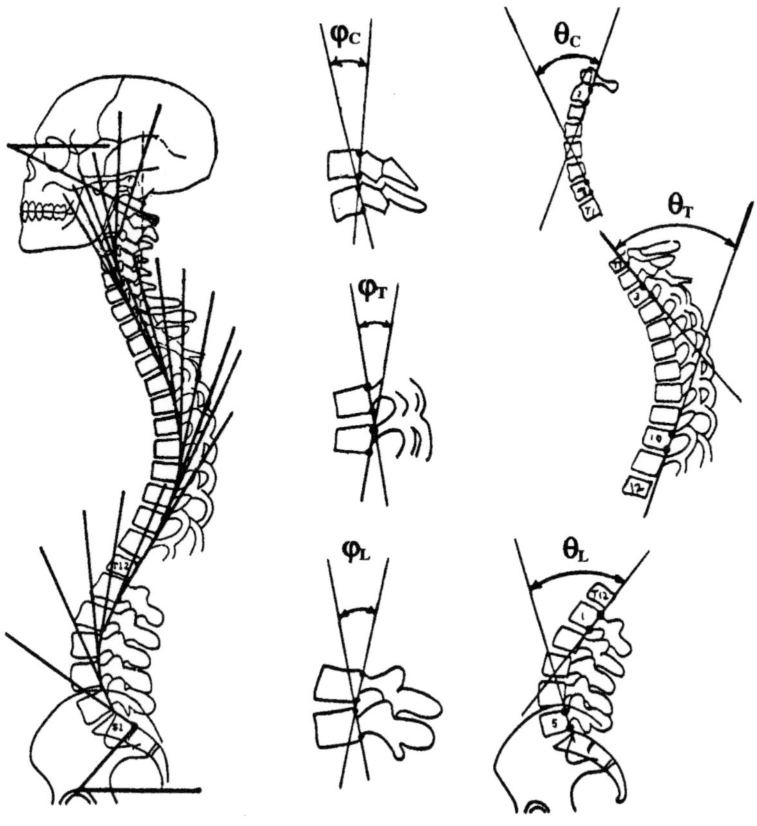

Figure 2.
Harrison posterior tangent method involves lines drawn contiguous with the posterior vertebral body margins. Intersegmental as well as regional sagittal curves are easily quantified having a standard error of measurement within about 2° (Courtesy CBP seminars).

been done [40, 41, 43–46]. The statistical differentiation of asymptomatic subjects from symptomatic pain group patients based on alignment data have been performed [42, 47]. The demonstration of paralleled spine alignment improvements with reduction in pain and disability, versus no change in untreated control groups in pre-post clinical trials have been performed [54–59]. The demonstration in randomized clinical trials that only patient groups achieving lordosis improvement (lumbar or cervical) and hyper-kyphosis (thoracic) reduction achieve long-term improvements in various outcome measures versus comparative treatment control groups not getting spine alignment improvement who experience regression in multiple outcome measures at follow-up have also been done [10–16, 60–64].

Chiropractors practicing Chiropractic BioPhysics® (CBP®) structural rehabilitation techniques have used this spine model as the goal of care for over 20 years; and more recently physical therapists and other manual medicine rehabilitation specialists have adopted components of this system as well. It is noted that this model serves as the baseline for patient comparison; specific patient comparisons, however, must include patient-specific considerations related to thoracic inlet parameters [65] as well as pelvic morphology [66] as these may dictate a structural modification to the model for a given patient. There are software programs (i.e. PostureRay Inc., Trinity FL, USA) that aid in the ability for practitioners to assess spine alignment quickly in daily practice (**Figure 3**). It must also be mentioned

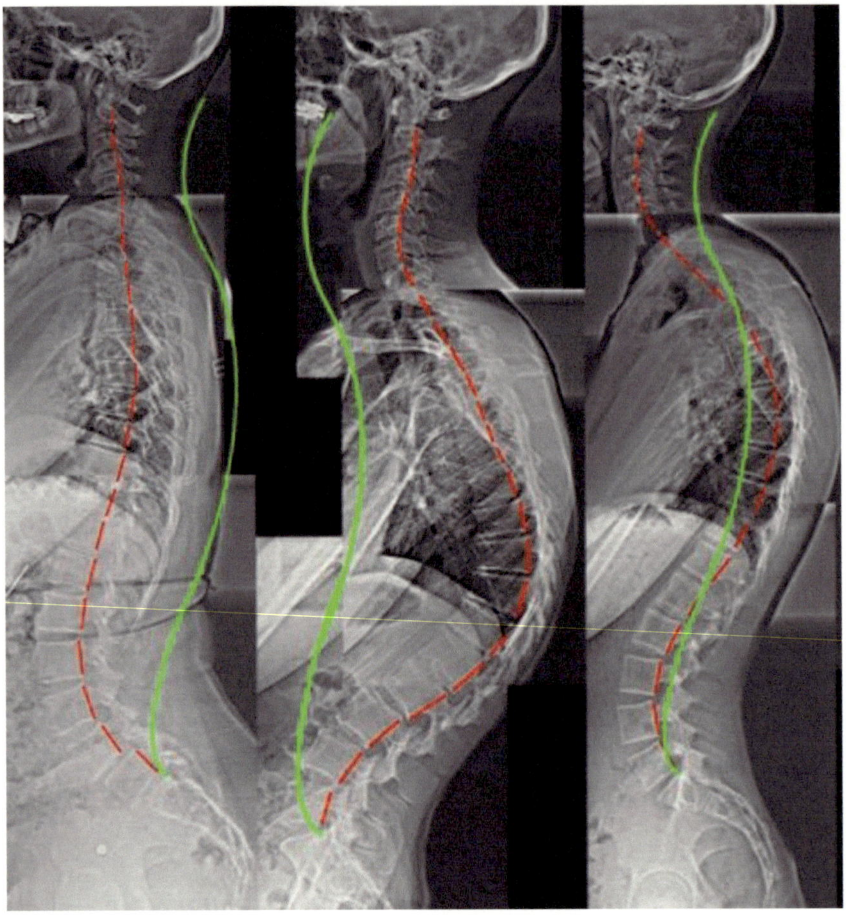

Figure 3.
Three patients demonstrating dramatically different spine alignment patterns. Left: Excessive lumbar hyperlordosis, L4 anterolisthesis, and excessive anterior sagittal balance in a mid-aged female with disabling low back pain; Middle: Excessive thoracolumbar kyphosis and early degenerative changes in a mid-aged male; Right: Excessive thoracic hyperkyphosis in a young male with Scheuermann's disease. Red line is contiguous with posterior vertebral body margins; green line represents Harrison normal spinal model (Courtesy PAO).

that proper assessment of the spine includes the whole spine, that is, the cervical, thoracic and lumbar regions and femur heads. This is because spine balance and compensation mechanisms involve the whole spine; thus, regional X-rays to the 'problem area' can mislead treatment and not account for distal spinopelvic compensations that need to be considered prior to initiating a trial of spine care by these methods.

3. Biomechanics of the central nervous system

The brainstem (mesencephalon, pons, medulla oblongata), cranial nerves V-XII, spinal cord, cauda equina, and nerve roots may collectively be referred to as the pons-cord tissue tract. The static and dynamic characteristics of the pons-cord tract constitutes a self-contained compartment of biomechanics [8, 9, 67]. This results from the way the cord is maintained within the canal by its many attachments: from above (being continuous with the brainstem), from below (sacral and coccyx attachment through the cauda equina and filum terminale), as well as throughout its length (intermittent dural attachments to the posterior longitudinal ligament, ventral attachments of the nerve root sleeves exiting the intervertebral foramina, and bilateral dentate ligament attachments ranging from the upper cervical region down to the level of L1). Under relatively normal static posture without pathological processes, spine dynamics produce normal or 'physiologic' tension as transmitted by its constraining elements, and without neurological compromise (**Figure 4**) [8, 9, 68].

Only when normal neurodynamic aspects of the so-called pons-cord tract are understood can neuropathology from adverse tensions be fully understood. As Breig states "Internal deformation of the tissue cannot be ruled out as a factor in any disease of the nervous system even in inflammatory and degenerative conditions of the hindbrain, cord and associated nerves, and in some cases it will be of primary pathologic significance" [8] (p. 12). A key concept is that under normal circumstances, normal movements of the spine involve physiologic unfolding and folding of the cord and nerve roots. Head flexion causes instantaneous unfolding and normal elasticity of the neural tissues and head extension causes elastic rebound and a re-folding of the cord and nerve roots (**Figure 4**). In this way the CNS can preserve normal function while accommodating differing spinal positions. Breig also found that movements of the cord occur at the location of movement as well as throughout the entire pons-cord tract; cervical motions produce strains (deformations) caudally down to the cauda equina and movements of the lower spine cause strains as far up as the cervical cord and brainstem. In fact, deformation of the brain tissue below the tentorium (which can affect cranial nerves V-XII [8]) within the cerebellum occurs to accommodate spine movements (particularly maximal functional positions).

All ventral flexion movements throughout the spine (i.e. cervical, thoracic, lumbar) cause a lengthening of the spinal canal, and therefore, a transmission of axial tension onto the cord. Pathological processes, such as disc herniations and bone spurs, if severe enough, interfere with the pons-cord tract biomechanics [69, 70], where the normal tension transmitted by the pons-cord restraining elements may then be referred to as 'pathological' tension [71]. Independent but equally as significant, abnormal spinal postures may create adverse tension within the neural elements as well. For instance, Stein found that "in a deformed kyphotic cervical spine, even a 'normal' amount of movement in the cervical spine may cause compression of the spinal cord" [72]. This is because the spinal cord adopts the length of the bony canal [73].

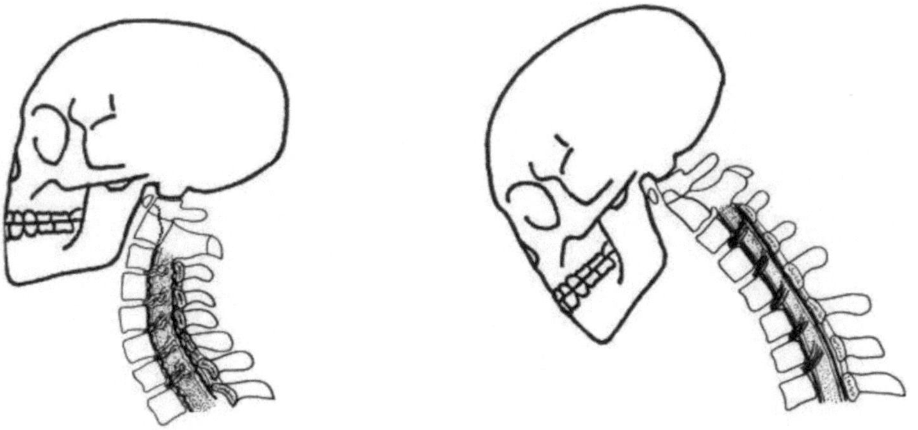

Figure 4.
Left: Physiologic folding of the cord and nerve roots in normal lordosis. Right: A forward flexion in those with normal lordosis causes normal unfolding and elasticity of the pons, cord and nerve roots that remain 'physiologic' or within tolerable tensions that do not overload the nervous system (Courtesy CBP Seminars).

Further, as suggested by Harrison et al. [74] static neutral postures or dynamically adopted combinations of postures; that is, rotations and translations of the head, thorax, or pelvis (**Figures 5** and **6**) [36], exert larger stresses and strains onto the pons-cord tissue tract. Thus, it can be deduced that the combination of pathological processes (bone spurs, disc herniations, etc.) and aberrations in posture (forward head posture, thoracic hyperkyphosis, etc.) may disrupt normal CNS biomechanics, and at levels below that at which either factor acting alone would elicit neurological symptoms. As it can be presumed when a patient has an accumulation of forward flexed spine positions, such as severe thoracic hyperkyphosis (THK) posture for example, the amount of spinal canal lengthening can be great and supersede the 'normal' or physiologic amount of unfolding and elastic deformation available within the pons-cord system. In this situation, normal physiologic tensions transition to become pathologic tensions causing intermittent over-stretching and over-straining of the tissues and ultimately, causing or exacerbating neurologic symptoms.

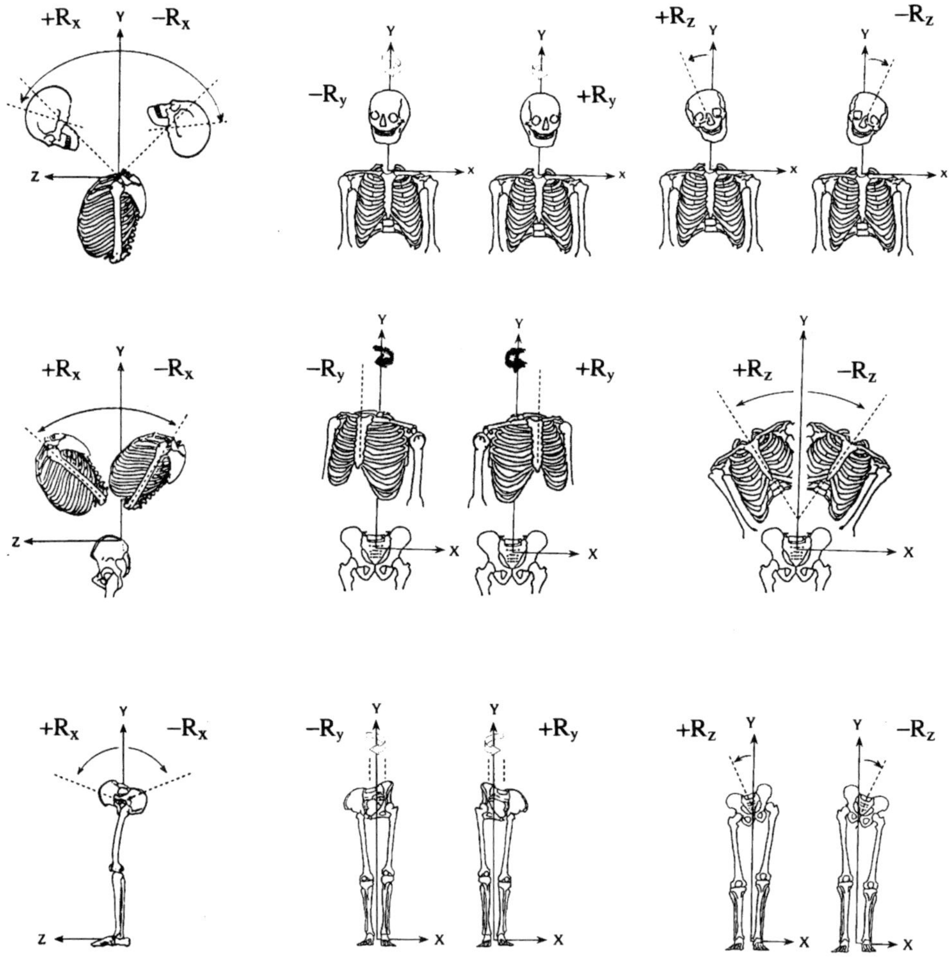

Figure 5.
If the head, thoracic cage, and pelvis are considered rigid bodies, then the possible rotations in 3-dimensions are illustrated. Flexion and extension are rotations on the x-axis, axial rotation is about the y-axis, and lateral flexion is rotation about the z-axis (Courtesy CBP Seminars).

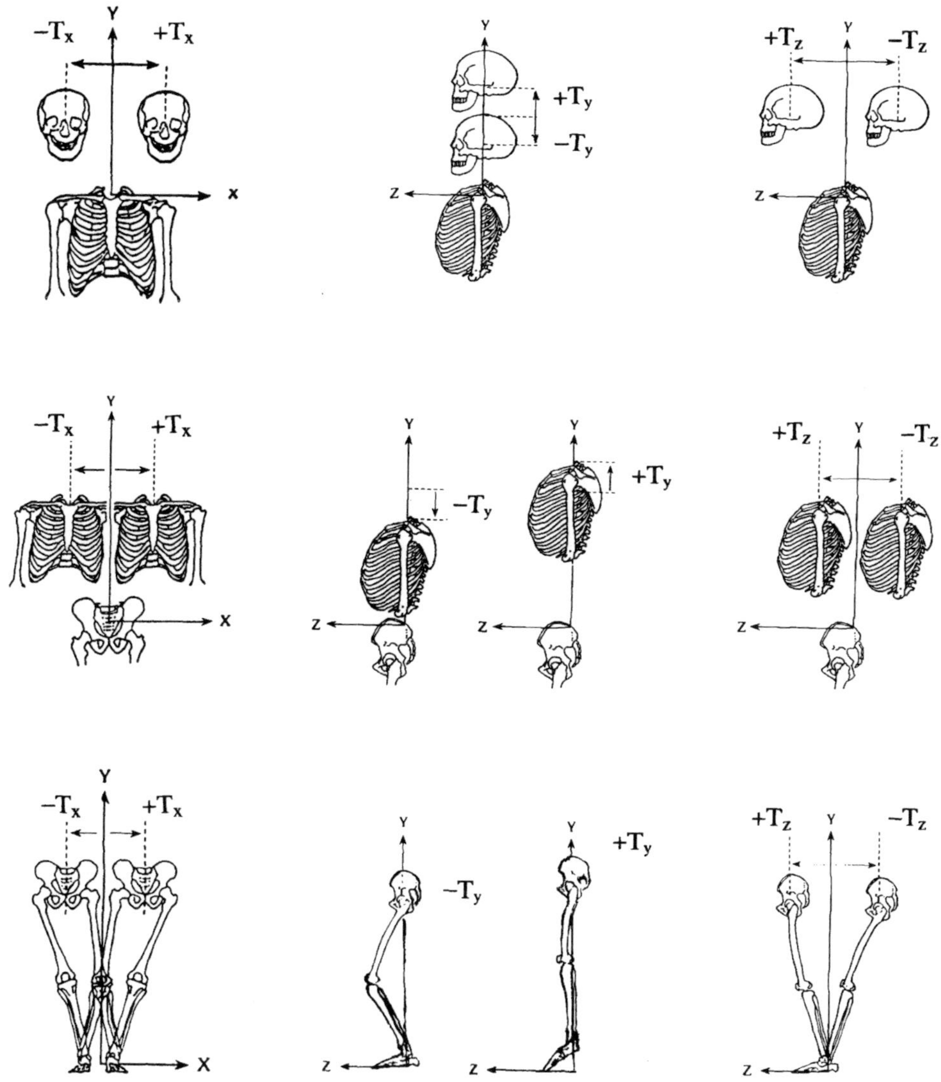

Figure 6.
If the head, thoracic cage, and pelvis are considered rigid bodies, then the possible translations in 3-dimensions are illustrated. Lateral translations occur along the x-axis, vertical translations occur along the y-axis, and anterior–posterior translations (protraction-retraction) occurs along the z-axis (Courtesy CBP Seminars).

4. Pathophysiologic mechanisms from adverse CNS tension

Understanding the normal biomechanics of the CNS lays the foundation for the understanding of postural-induced neurological signs and symptoms. As discussed, two main events may individually, or in combination, lead to excessive stresses (longitudinal, torsional, pure bending, shear) and strains (longitudinal cross-sectional) that are sufficient to produce symptoms. In words, poor postures (lengthened spinal canal via forward flexed spinal positions) and space occupying lesions (bone spurs, intervertebral disc prolapse, etc.) combine to produce symptomatology. The greater the spinal canal is flexed, or as discussed, the presence of combinations of rotations and translations in posture, the greater the forced unfolding and elastically stretched pons-cord tract (**Figure** 7). With the addition of space occupying lesions, patients having deviations in postural alignment become much more likely to succumb to various pressure mechanisms, or how the nervous tissue is compressed upon certain positions and movements.

It is important to realize that those patients with poor spinal posture may at times be in positions that are tolerable by the pons-cord tract (i.e. not over-stretched), and at other times perform movements that dynamically lengthen the spinal canal causing a pivotal transition to over-stress and over-strain the system (i.e. dynamic stress and strain). Therefore, successful symptomatic relief resulting from postural correction to a patient suffering from neurological complaints may be elucidated. Although some spinal pathologies will not change (e.g. bone spurs), the reduction of forward flexion of the neutral postural position (e.g. increasing cervical/lumbar hypo-lordosis; reducing thoracic hyper-kyphosis) will change the resting, and therefore the dynamic tensions throughout the pons-cord tract sufficiently enough to reduce the tensions from surpassing some pathological tension threshold (maintaining physiologic or normal tensions), and therefore alleviate neurologic symptomatology [74, 75].

How does adverse mechanical tensions within the CNS produce symptoms? Ultimately, pathological CNS tensions affect the vascular supply and therefore the perfusion of the neural tissues or they may affect the actual nerve conduction ability of the nerve cells (causing hyper or hypo function). Mathematically, perfusion = mean arteriole pressure (MAP) – cord interstitial pressure (CIP) [76]. Thus, for perfusion to remain adequate, the MAP must remain greater than CIP. However, as discussed by Harrison et al. [77], an increase in CIP can be caused by at least two forces, a longitudinal force causing unfolding and elastic elongation of the cord, and a transverse force usually by the cord being thrust into the posterior margin of the vertebral body at the anterior portion of the spinal canal. As stated, Stein found that cervical kyphosis, posture subluxation alone is enough to interfere with cord conduction [72], but with an accompanying space occupying lesion the likelihood for a transverse cord/nerve compression pressure mechanism to limit perfusion and compromise neural function is much greater.

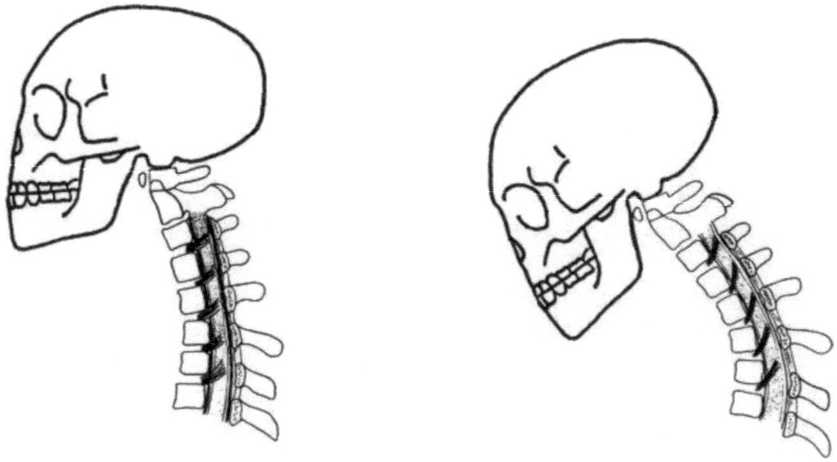

Figure 7.
Left: Cervical kyphosis subluxation in neutral posture results in the unfolding and elastic pre-tension present prior to flexion. Right: Forward flexion of a kyphotic neck may result in 'pathologic' or pons-cord-nerve root tensions that exceed physiologic limits and results in neurologic symptoms; particularly in the presence of a space-occupying lesion such as a bone spur or intervertebral disc prolapse (Courtesy CBP Seminars).

5. Postural correction to treat neurologic disorders by reducing pons-cord tensions

There have been several clinical controlled trials documenting the association with improved postural parameters (e.g. increasing cervical lordosis, increasing lumbar lordosis, decreasing thoracic hyperkyphosis) translating into improved physiological measures including specific tests indicative of neurologic function [10–16]. These measures include:

- Central somatosensory conduction time N13-N20 (**Figure 8**);
- Dermatomal somatosensory evoked potentials (DSSEPs) (**Figures 9** and **10**);
- H-reflex;
- Sensorimotor control measures (**Figures 11** and **12**);
- Sympathetic skin resistance response (**Figure 13**).

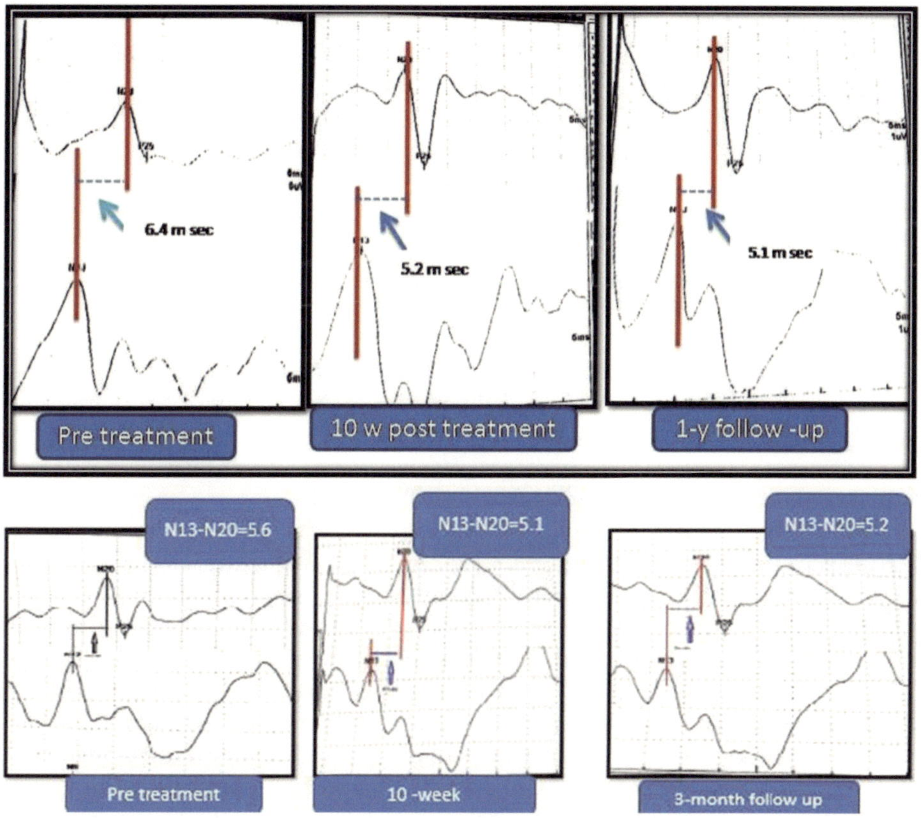

Figure 8.
Central conduction time (N13-N20) also known as spinal cord velocity. In the top figure, a representative example of central conduction time (N13-N20) at three intervals of measurement: baseline, following 10-weeks of treatment, and 1-year follow-up. This is from the study by Moustafa et al. [13] on symptomatic patients with cervical spine disc herniation. Follow correction of the cervical lordosis, a 20% change in central conduction speed is shown in milliseconds (m sec) indicating a faster more efficient response. In the bottom graph a representative sample from the study of Moustafa et al. [78] is shown. Here, in asymptomatic participants, correction of the cervical lordosis and anterior head posture was found to result in a 10% faster response in the central conduction time potential. Comparative and placebo control groups not attaining spine correction showed no improvement in central conduction time.

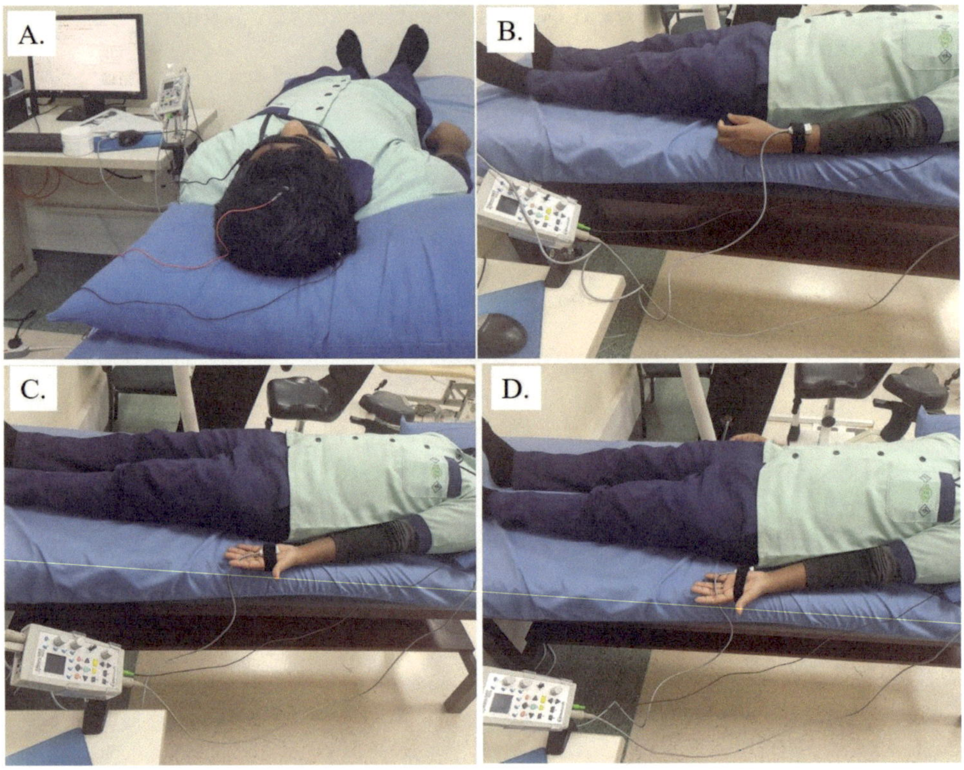

Figure 9.
Dermatomal somatosensory evoked potential (DSSEPs) set up for C6, C7, and C8 nerve root assessment. In (A) Sites of recording: (1) active recording electrode at c3', (2) reference electrode at Fz, and (3) grounding electrode at Fbz. Location of stimulation sites are indicated above: (B) for C6 dermatome, (C) for C7 dermatome, (D) C8 dermatome. Sites of recording. Courtesy of Moustafa et al. [16].

Here we briefly summarize the particulars of exemplary trials that demonstrate how improvement in targeted spinal and postural parameters have led to improved neurophysiological outcomes.

5.1 Central somatosensory conduction time N13-N20

Using standardized clinical procedures for median nerve stimulation at the wrist, a subjects' central somatosensory conduction time measurement, N13-N20, can be determined. Differences in peak latencies between N13 and N20 is measured as central conduction time or similarly called 'cervical spinal cord velocity'. In 2016, Moustafa et al. reported on a randomized controlled trial using a cervical extension traction orthotic device (Denneroll™; Denneroll Ptdy, limited, Sydney, Australia) in a multimodal rehabilitation program for treating patients with discogenic radiculopathy [13]. Sixty patients were randomized to a treatment and comparison (control) group where both groups received TENS, thoracic spine manipulation, soft tissue mobilization and strengthening exercises. Only the treatment group performed the additional Denneroll orthotic device to increase cervical lordosis and reduce forward head posture. After 30 treatment applications over the course of 10-weeks, only the treatment group demonstrated significant improvements in N13-N20 (20% gain in velocity). Also, at a 1-year follow-up without further intervention, again only the treatment group demonstrated a statistically improved N13-N20 potential. Importantly, only the treatment group receiving the Denneroll had statistically improved cervical lordosis and reduced forward head posture at the 10-week and 1-year follow-up. **Figure 8** (top) demonstrates the improvement in the N13-N20 potential in this trial.

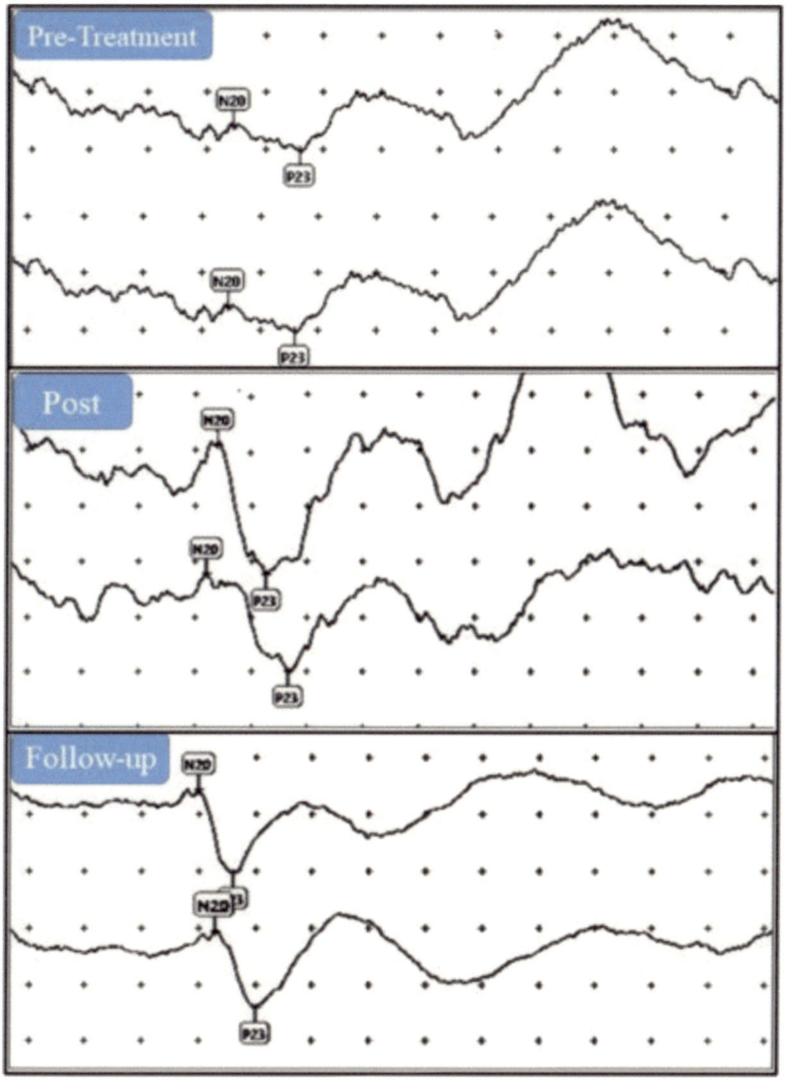

Figure 10.
Example of Dermatomal somatosensory evoked potential (DSSEPs) of C6 dermatome at three intervals of measurement. Courtesy of Moustafa et al. [16]. The Pre-treatment DSSEPs from the RCT by Moustafa et al. [16] is shown. In the 10-week post treatment (Follow-up), the DSSEPs following cervical curve correction is shown. Finally, the 3-month (Post) follow-up, DSSEPs are shown where correction was stable over time.

In another trial, Moustafa et al. reported on the unique treatment of asymptomatic volunteers who had strictly defined anterior head translation and cervical hypolordosis [78]. Eighty persons were randomized into a treatment group who performed cervical extension traction on the Denneroll traction orthotic or a control group who lied on a rolled hydrocollator towel (placebo control). Both groups were treated for 30 sessions over 10-weeks and were then re-assessed after 12 further weeks of no further treatment. Central somatosensory conduction time latency (N13-N20) and amplitudes of spinal (N13), brainstem (P14), parietal (N20 and P27), and frontal (N30) potentials were measured at baseline (prior to treatment), 10-weeks and 22-weeks. After the 10-weeks of treatment, the treatment group had significantly better amplitudes of N13, P14, N20, N27 and N30 as well as central conduction time (10% faster conduction velocity of N13-N20). All significant differences between groups favouring the treatment group remained at the 12-week post-treatment follow-up. Lastly, a statistically significant multiple

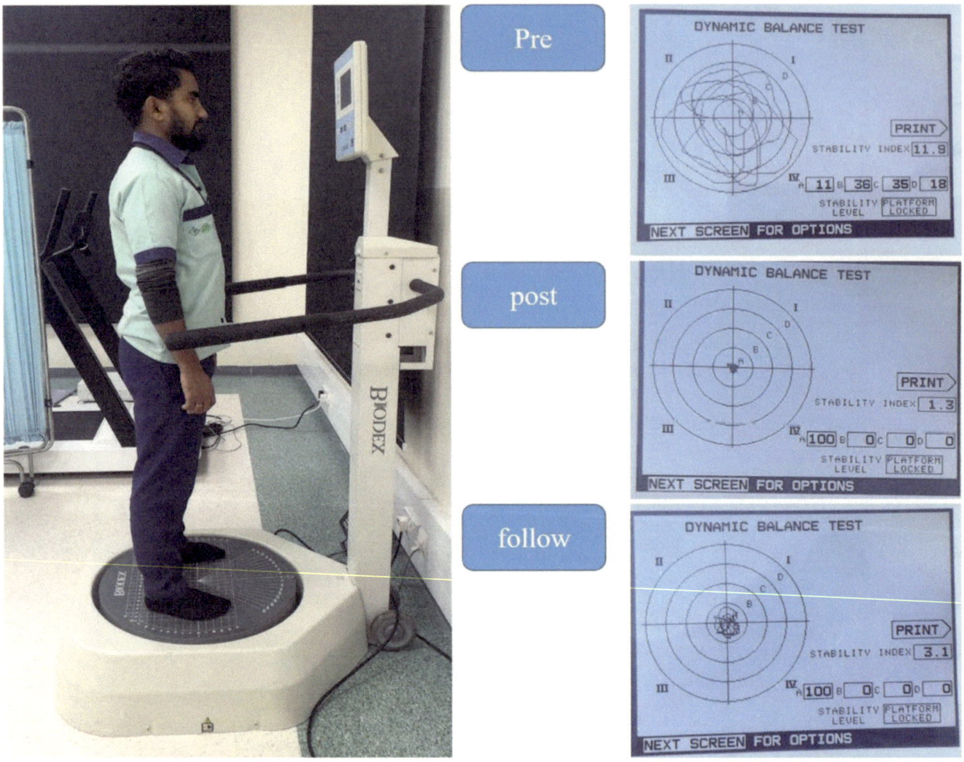

Figure 11.
Postural stability characteristics were evaluated with a Biodex Balance System SD (BBS) (Biodex Medical Systems, Inc., Shirley, NY). Dynamic balance testing was performed on the unlocked platform to allow free movement concurrently both in the anterior–posterior (AP) and medial-lateral (ML) directions. The platform permits variable levels of resistance to movement perturbation ranging from one to eight (1 being the most restrictive). BBS measures the deviation of each axis during dynamic balance assessments. The BBS software measures an overall stability index (OSI) and is a representative index of balance performance. OSI is the best indicator of the overall ability of the subject to balance the platform whereby a reduced balance or stability correlates with large variation or large value of OSI [79] [80]. From the RCT by Moustafa et al. [10] participants randomized to and achieving cervical spine correction obtained statistically significant improvements in the OSI compared to a standard care group (Pre vs. 10-weeks post vs. 1-year follow up). Courtesy of Moustafa et al. [10, 34].

regression model to predict central conduction time changes, N13-N20, from correction in cervical lordosis and anterior head translation (AHT) was identified for the intervention group receiving the Denneroll orthotic at both the 10-week mark ($p < .001$) and the 3-month follow-up ($p < .001$) [78]. **Figure 8** (bottom) demonstrates the improvement in the N13-N20 potential in this trial.

5.2 Dermatomal somatosensory evoked potentials (DSSEPs)

In 2011, Moustafa et al. reported on the results of a pilot trial that showed patients with cervical spondylotic radiculopathy randomized to a rehabilitation program including cervical spine stretching exercises, infrared radiation and 3-point bending cervical extension traction had significantly improved peak-to-peak amplitude measures of DSSEPs after both 10-weeks of treatment (30 treatment sessions) and at a 12-week follow-up [16]. The comparison (control) group receiving the same treatment less the neck traction did show an initial improvement in DSSEPs after the 10-week treatment period, however, this difference disappeared at the 12-week follow-up. Only the treatment group showed a statistically significant increase in cervical lordosis. Most importantly, Moustafa et al. identified a linear correlation between initial

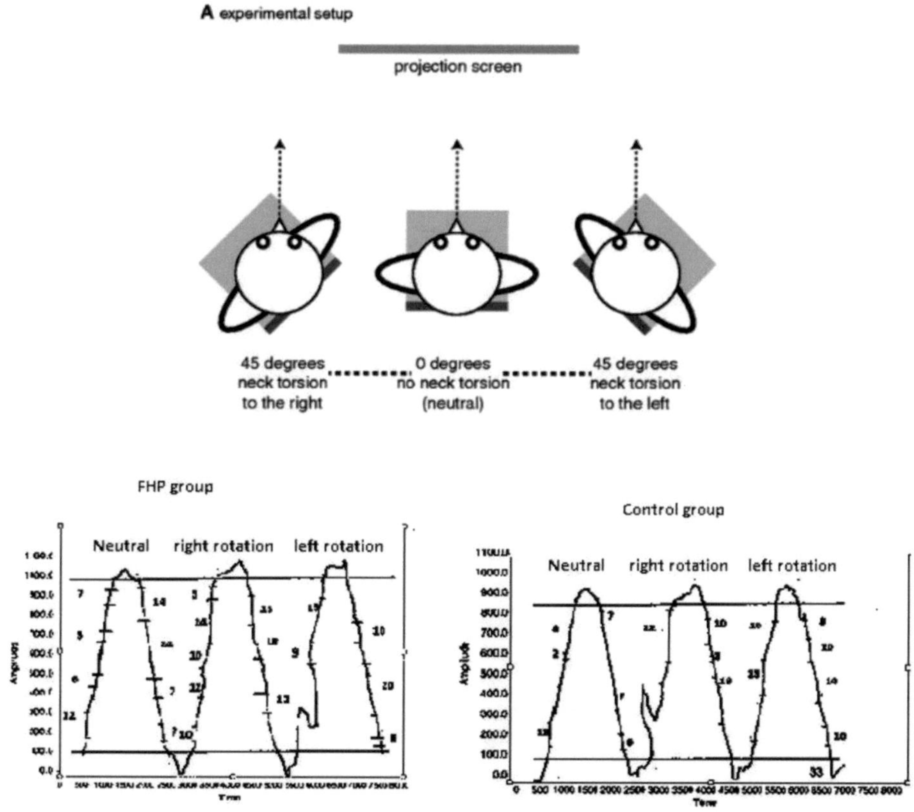

Figure 12.
In A, an example of the smooth pursuit neck torsion test (SPNT) is shown neutral, right turn, and left turn of the head indicated by the 45° torso rotated position. Middle and right image: A SPNT test eye velocity is shown as the uneven high amplitude curves. The ciphers indicate the length of the vertical part of the curve between two marks, i.e., the saccades. The forward head posture group (FHP group) has larger errors (≈30%) as compared to a match control group with normal head alignment (10% average error). Courtesy of Moustafa et al. [34].

DSSEPs and cervical lordosis magnitude for both groups ($r = .65$; $p < 0.0001$), whereas this relationship was only maintained in the study group receiving 2-way traction at final follow-up ($r = .55$; $p = 0.033$). This indicates that cervical spine lordotic correction linearly correlates to improvements in DSSEPs [16]. **Figures 9** and **10** depict the experimental setup for the DSSEPs of C6, C7, and C8 as well as the changes in C6 DSSEPs in the study group receiving the curve corrective traction.

As reported in the previous section (5.1), the 2016 trial reported by Moustafa et al. [13] treating patients with discogenic radiculopathy, both groups showed improvements in latency of DSSEPs at the 10-week post-treatment assessments, however only the treatment group showed statistically improved amplitude of DSSEPs. At a 1-year follow-up without intervention, only the treatment group demonstrated statistically improved latency and amplitude of DSSEPs. Also, only the treatment group had improved cervical lordosis and reduced forward head posture at the 10-week and 1-year follow-up.

5.3 H-reflex

In a unique randomized trial, Moustafa and colleagues [14] investigated the hypothesis that improving the cervical lordosis and reducing forward head translation would improve low back pain, disability, and neurophysiology in a sample of

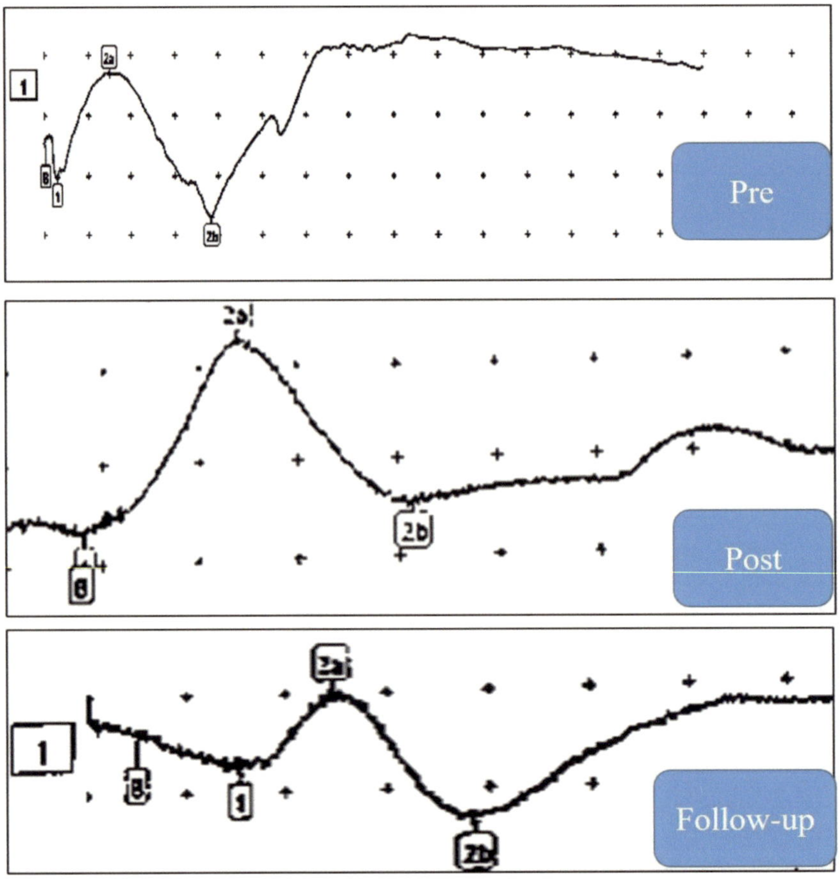

Figure 13.
Sympathetic skin resistance response (SSR). For measurement of the SSR, EMG equipment was used [10]. Active surface electrodes were attached on the palmar side, and the references were placed on the dorsum of the hand. The stimulus was given at the wrist contralateral to the recording side. Measurements were taken from left and right arms. Latencies were measured from the stimulation artifact to the first deflection from the baseline. The amplitude is measured from the peak of the first deflection to the peak of the next one (peak to peak) as shown. Depicted are the results for the study group receiving cervical spine correction (lordosis and forward head posture). On the Top: the study group receiving spine corrective extension traction is shown at pre-study; Middle: after 10 weeks of treatment (30 sessions); and Bottom: at 1-year follow up with no further treatment. Only the group receiving extension traction obtained sagittal plane cervical correction and statistically significant improvement in SSR latency and amplitude. Courtesy of Moustafa et al. [10].

80 (35 female) patients between 40 and 55 years suffering signs and symptoms from chronic discogenic lumbar radiculopathy (CDLR). Both groups received TENS therapy and hot packs; additionally, the study group received the Denneroll cervical traction orthotic. All treatment interventions were applied at a frequency of 3 x per week for 10 weeks. Both groups were followed for 6 months after their 10-week re-evaluation. Statistically significant differences between the study groups and the control group's postural measures were found favouring improved posture in the Denneroll group for: lumbar lordotic curve ($p = .002$), thoracic kyphosis ($p = .001$), trunk inclination ($p = .01$) and imbalance ($p = .001$), pelvic inclination ($p = .005$), and surface rotation ($p = 0.01$). The two radiographic measures of cervical lordosis ($p = .001$) and forward head posture ($p = .002$), and H reflex amplitude ($p = .007$) and H reflex latency ($p = .001$) were likewise statistically different between the groups at 10 weeks favoring improvement in the Denneroll study group. Restoring cervical lordosis and reduction of forward head posture with Denneroll traction was found to have a positive impact on 3D posture parameters, leg and back pain

scores, back disability, and H reflex latency and amplitude. Thus, improvement of sagittal cervical spine posture and alignment benefited the pain, disability, and postural imbalances in patients with CDLR.

In 2013, Moustafa et al. reported the results of a trial employing lumbar extension traction to increase the lumbar lordosis in patients suffering from MRI-verified lumbosacral radiculopathy [15]. Sixty-four patients were randomly allocated to the treatment or comparison (control) group who both received hot packs and interferential therapy; only the treatment group received the lumbar extension traction. After 30 treatment sessions over 10-weeks, only the treatment group showed statistically improved latency and amplitude of the H-reflex. At the 6-month follow-up, again, only the treatment group showed statistically improved H-reflex outcomes. Only the treatment group demonstrated improved lumbar lordosis after the 10-week treatment period and at the 6-month follow-up.

5.4 Sensorimotor control measures

5.4.1 Cervicocephalic kinesthetic sense measured as head repositioning accuracy

Improvement in head repositioning accuracy (HRA) as a result of sagittal plane spine alignment correction has been assessed in three recent randomized trials by the Moustafa et al. group; two of these trials assessed cervical lordotic correction and anterior head translation reduction [10, 79], whereas, one trial assessed improvement in thoracic hyper-kyphosis [11]. In 2017, Moustafa et al. reported on the improvement in HRA, a measurement of cervicocephalic kinesthetic sensibility [79]. Seventy-two patients suffering from cervicogenic dizziness were randomized to a treatment or comparison (control) group and received TENS, hot packs, mobilization, myofascial and suboccipital release, and therapeutic functional exercises. Only the treatment group also received the Denneroll cervical extension traction orthotic device. The cervical range of motion (CROM) device was used to assess cervicocephalic kinesthetic sensibility by measuring the head repositioning average error (*HRA*). The participants (blindfolded) started with their head in the neutral head position (NHP) and were asked to actively move to the midpoint of their maximum rotation range, which was called the "target position." After returning to the NHP, they were then asked to rotate their head to the target position. The difference between the target position and the achieved position was recorded 3 times and averaged. The midpoint position was used rather than the NHP because it was considered a non-learned position. The CROM device has good criterion validity (r = 0.89–0.99) and reliability (intra-class correlation coefficient [ICC] = 0.92–0.96) [80].

After 30 treatment session over 10-weeks, both groups improved on the HRA test [79]. However, at the 1-year follow-up, the treatment group's HRA to the left and right was statistically significantly better than the comparison group. Again, only the treatment group had a statistically improved cervical lordosis and improved forward head posture at both the 10-week and 1-year follow-up. In their more recent [10] randomized trial similar results were identified where improved HRA resulted from improved cervical lordosis and forward head translation reduction; herein, the improvement in the HRA was identified to be linearly correlated to the improvement in both cervical lordosis and reduction in forward head posture. The linear correlation between improved HRA and improved forward head posture magnitude is further supported by the results of a cross-sectional case control investigation which found a linear relationship between worsening HRA and increased magnitudes of forward head posture [34].

In 2020, Moustafa et al. reported on the improvements in various sensorimotor control measures in patients treated for thoracic hyper-kyphosis [11]. Eighty patients with thoracic hyper-kyphosis were randomized to a treatment or comparison (control) group. Both groups were treated for 30 treatment sessions over a 10-week time period with TENS and hot packs, soft tissue mobilization, thoracic spine manipulation, and functional exercises. Only the treatment group also performed the Denneroll thoracic traction orthotic designed to reduce the thoracic curve. At the 10-week post-treatment assessment, no significant differences were found for left-sided HRA whereas, significant differences favouring the treatment group were found for the right sided HRA. At the 1-year follow-up without intervention, sensorimotor control measurement of HRA, bilaterally, was significantly superior for the intervention group. Also, only the treatment group experienced a reduction in thoracic hyper-kyphosis at the 10-week assessment that was maintained at the 1-year follow-up [11].

5.4.2 Biodex balance and stability measurement

Posture stability efficiency is a key measurement or performance variable of sensorimotor control. In recent randomized trials [10, 11] and case control [34] investigations by Moustafa and colleagues, postural stability characteristics were evaluated with a Biodex Balance System SD (BBS) (Biodex Medical Systems, Inc., Shirley, NY) (**Figure 11**). Dynamic balance testing was performed on the unlocked platform to allow free movement concurrently in both the anterior–posterior (AP) and medial-lateral (ML) directions. The platform permits variable levels of resistance to movement perturbation ranging from one to eight (1 being the most restrictive). BBS measures the deviation of each axis during dynamic balance assessments. The BBS software measures an overall stability index (OSI) and is a representative index of balance performance. OSI is the best indicator of the overall ability of the subject to balance the platform whereby a reduced balance or stability correlates with large variation or large value of OSI [81, 82]. From the RCT by Moustafa et al. [10], participants randomized to and achieving correction of both cervical lordosis and anterior head posture obtained statistically significant improvements in the OSI compared to a standard care group (pre vs. 10-weeks post vs. 1-year follow up). Likewise, in the RCT looking at thoracic hyper-kyphosis reduction, it was found that OSI was statistically improved only in the group achieving reduction of thoracic kyphosis and that this result was stable at 1-year follow-up [11].

The fact that posture stability, as measured with OSI, improves due to correction of the sagittal cervical and thoracic spine alignments seems to make sense; as previously a linearly correlation between worsening OSI and increased magnitudes of forward head posture has been found [34].

5.4.3 Smooth pursuit neck torsion test or SPNT

The smooth pursuit neck torsion test (SPNT) is used to quantify alterations in and improvement in a person's visual-motor control using electro-oculography equipment [83]. **Figure 12** demostrates the SPNT procedure. First, participants perform the SPNT with the head and trunk in the neutral, forward facing posture. Next, while keeping the head facing forward, the torso is placed in a 45° rotation (about a vertical y-axis) position to each side in a consecutive manner. Participants typically perform three blinks of their eyes and are instructed to follow the path of a light source as close as possible with their eyes without movement of their head or neck. The accuracy of the SPNT is determined as the difference between the average increase/decrease in the participants NHP vs. the torsioned positions; errors are termed 'corrective saccades' and are reported as a percentage difference from perfect. In a recent case control cohort sample, Moustafa et al. [34] identified that the forward head posture group (FHP group) had larger SPNT errors (≈30%) as compared to a matched control group with normal head alignment (10% average error). In fact, a linear correlation was identified between the magnitude of forward head posture subluxation and the percent error in SPNT.

Importantly, in the Moustafa et al. RCTs [10, 11], SPNT test eye velocity was shown to improve in the group receiving spine correction as compared to the comparison group not receiving and not achieving spine correction. The average SPNT errors in both the cervical spine [10] and the thoracic spine [11] correction groups improved down to bench-mark values for healthy persons (≈10%).

5.5 Dysafferentation, altered sensorimotor control and autonomic nervous system

Sympathetic skin resistance response (SSR) is a measurement of autonomic nervous system function or dysfunction. For measurement of the SSR, EMG equipment is typically used [10, 34]. Active surface electrodes are attached on the palmar side, and the references are placed on the dorsum of the hand. A stimulus is given at the wrist contralateral to the recording side. Measurements should typically be taken from left and right arms. The SSR is assessed as: (1) a latency measurement from the stimulation artifact to the first deflection from the baseline; and (2) an amplitude is measured from the peak of the first deflection to the peak of the next one (peak to peak). **Figure 13** depicts a typical measurement of SSR latency and amplitude.

In a recent case–control cohort investigation of 160 asymptomatic volunteers, Moustafa and colleagues [34] investigated the SSR and its relationship to the severity of forward head posture; a strong linear correlation was identified between the magnitude of forward head posture and increased amplitude and latency of the SSR evoked potentials. Thus, increased magnitudes of forward head posture have a negative impact on the autonomic nervous system in essence leading to a state of hyperactivity or increased excitability. Only one RCT on the effects of spine correction on SSR latency and amplitude could be identified. In the study by Moustafa et al. [10], the group receiving spine corrective extension traction obtained sagittal plane cervical correction and statistically significant improvement in SSR latency and amplitude; the results indicated a linear correlation between the amount of correction of the cervical lordosis and FHP and the concomitant improvement of the SSR potentials [10].

6. Strengths, applications, and perspectives

The above review of sagittal plane spine alignment and its impact on neurophysiology has several strengths. First, there is strong biomechanical evidence indicating that altered and sustained sagittal plane spine and posture alignment results in increasing the stresses and strains acting on the pons-cord tract system and that this impairs directly or indirectly neurophysiology; this evidence has existed since 1960 [8, 9, 26, 68, 69, 71–75, 77]. Second, considering the results of the recent randomized trials reviewed above, it is clear, that rehabilitation techniques that increase the cervical lordosis and lumbar lordosis, have a profound and sustained effect of improving measurements of neurophysiology as measured with DSSEP's, H-Reflex, and central conduction times [12–16, 78, 79]. Similarly, reducing the magnitudes of thoracic hyper-kyphosis [11] and FHP [12–16, 78, 79] has been found in RCT's to result in improved neurophysiological measurements. Finally, clinical management and improvement of several complex neurological disorders have been documented in multiple case reports where spine correction was suggested to be the important variable which improved the patient's neurophysiological disorder [17–25]. Thus, considering the facts that biomechanics studies, randomized trials, and case reports all point to the same finding, clinically and scientifically one would need to concede that improved neurophysiology following correction of the abnormal spine towards normal values is an evidence-based and logical approach to pursue with appropriate patients.

Similarly, the known intimate connections between afferent input (from the proprioceptive, visual and vestibular systems) and stable upright postures of the head and neck [28] and the fact that there exists a plethora of mechanoreceptors in the cervical spine soft tissues providing necessary neurophysiological input in a feed forward and feedback system provides a strong fundamental physiological basis for the concept that altered spine alignment can have a profound effect on sensorimotor control via connections to the vestibular, visual and central nervous systems [29]. Furthermore, and as explicitly stated in the introduction to this chapter, a complex network of neurophysiological connections between cervical spine mechanoreceptors and the sympathetic nervous system exists [30–32]. This information coupled with the findings of both case control investigations [34] and randomized trials [10, 11, 63, 79] provides strong clinical evidence that restoring normal sagittal plane posture and cervical spine alignment is important for a better afferentation process, improved sensorimotor control, and improved autonomic nervous system function.

Clinically, the astute reader should recognize the need to radiographically assess the full spine alignment, in particular the sagittal plane, to identify if a patient is a candidate and in need of true spine correction; that is, structural rehabilitation of the spine and posture. A comparison of the patient's spine and posture should be made against tested normal alignment values such as the Harrison full spine model and posture displacement models discussed herein. Furthermore, the addition of fundamental neurophysiological testing and the basic parts of sensorimotor control measurements should be considered as important assessments during patient evaluations. Once an indication for corrective care has been identified, the clinical administration of specific spine mirror image corrective exercises and extension traction methods should be employed. Previously, we have discussed the techniques, indications and contraindications, timing of, and applications for several known spine corrective methods and the clinician should be willing to add these to their armamentarium for patient care; we refer the reader to this source [35]. Adding the goal and methods of true spine correction to the clinical outcomes of patient care should not be foreign, it should not be in disregard to traditional strength and functional conditioning; it should simply be part of the basic, fundamental treatment approach for abnormalities of the human frame in the effort to improve a variety of spine related and neurophysiological disorders.

7. Conclusion

This chapter has explored the hypothesis and evidence that restoring normal posture and spine alignment has important influences on neurophysiology, sensorimotor control and autonomic nervous system functionality. There is limited but high-quality research identifying that sagittal spine alignment restoration plays an important role in improving neurophysiology, sensorimotor control, and autonomic nervous system function. Within the limitations of the fact that only a handful of clinical trials exist on the topics discussed in this chapter, the unique contribution and importance of this review is that it demonstrates that radiographic determined re-alignment of the sagittal spine and posture plays a significant role in long-term management outcomes in people suffering from a variety of musculoskeletal, and health related disorders. Improved neurophysiological function as measured via dermatomal somatosensory evoked potentials, spinal cord velocity (N13-N20 potential), sensorimotor control, and sympathetic nervous system activity is directly influenced by and improved by full spine sagittal alignment in general and, more specifically, to cervical posture and spine alignment. This review identifies main issues that warrant further investigations to elucidate primary interactions and to identify ideal populations that would benefit from structural rehabilitation of the spine and posture techniques as discussed herein.

Conflict of interest

PAO is a paid consultant to CBP; DEH teaches spine rehabilitation methods and sells products related to the treatment of spine deformities. IMM has nothing to declare.

Nomenclature

AP	Anterior–posterior
BBS	Biodex Balance System SD
CBP	Chiropractic BioPhysics®
CDLR	Chronic discogenic lumbar radiculopathy
CIP	Cord interstitial pressure
CNS	Central nervous system
CROM	Cervical range of motion
CSM	Cervical spondylotic myelopathy
CTS	Carpal tunnel syndrome
DSSEPs	Dermatomal somatosensory evoked potentials
EMG	Electromyography
FHP	Forward head posture
HRA	Head repositioning accuracy
MAP	Mean arteriole pressure
ML	Medial-lateral
MRI	Magnetic resonance imaging
NHP	Neutral head position
N13-N20	Central conduction time
OSI	Overall stability index
PD	Parkinson's disease
RCT	Randomized controlled trial
SPNT	Smooth pursuit neck torsion
SSR	Sympathetic skin resistance
TENS	Transcutaneous electrical nerve stimulation
THK	Thoracic hyper-kyphosis
TN	Trigeminal neuralgia
TS	Tourette's syndrome

Author details

Paul A. Oakley[1*], Ibrahim M. Moustafa[2,3] and Deed E. Harrison[4]

1 Private Practice, Newmarket, Ontario, Canada

2 Department of Physiotherapy, College of Health Sciences, University of Sharjah, Sharjah, UAE

3 Basic Science Department, Faculty of Physical Therapy, Cairo University, Naser City, Cairo, Egypt

4 CBP NonProfit, Inc., Eagle, Idaho, USA

*Address all correspondence to: docoakley.icc@gmail.com

References

[1] Le Huec JC, Thompson W, Mohsinaly Y, Barrey C, Faundez A. Sagittal balance of the spine. Eur Spine J. 2019 Sep;28(9):1889-1905.

[2] Shah AA, Lemans JV, Zavatsky J. Spinal Balance/Alignment - Clinical Relevance and Biomechanics. J Biomech Eng. 2019; May 2. doi: 10.1115/1.4043650. [Epub ahead of print]

[3] Ling FP, Chevillotte T, Leglise A, Thompson W, Bouthors C, Le Huec JC. Which parameters are relevant in sagittal balance analysis of the cervical spine? A literature review. Eur Spine J. 2018;27(Suppl 1):8-15.

[4] Patwardhan AG, Khayatzadeh S, Havey RM, Voronov LI, Smith ZA, Kalmanson O, Ghanayem AJ, Sears W. Cervical sagittal balance: a biomechanical perspective can help clinical practice. Eur Spine J. 2018;27(Suppl 1):25-38.

[5] Le Huec JC, Saddiki R, Franke J, Rigal J, Aunoble S. Equilibrium of the human body and the gravity line: the basics. Eur Spine J. 2011;20 Suppl 5:558-563.

[6] Roussouly P, Pinheiro-Franco JL. Biomechanical analysis of the spino-pelvic organization and adaptation in pathology. Eur Spine J. 2011;20 Suppl 5:609-618.

[7] Harrison DE, Harrison DD, Troyanovich SJ, Harmon S. A normal spinal position: It's time to accept the evidence. J Manipulative Physiol Ther. 2000;23:623-644.

[8] Breig A. Biomechanics of the central nervous system. Stockholm, Almquist & Wicksell, 1960.

[9] Breig A. Adverse mechanical tension in the central nervous system. Stockholm, Almquist & Wicksell, 1978.

[10] Moustafa IM et al. Demonstration of autonomic nervous system function and cervical sensorimotor control after cervical lordosis rehabilitation in patients with chronic nonspecific neck pain: A randomized controlled trial. J Athletic Training. 2021; In Press.

[11] Moustafa IM, Walton LM, Raigangir V, Shousha TM, Harrison D. Reduction of posture hyperkyphosis improves short- and long-term outcomes in patients with neck pain. Abstract In J Orthop Sports Phys Ther. 2020;50(1):CSM143.

[12] Moustafa IM, Diab AAM, Hegazy FA, Harrison DE. Does rehabilitation of cervical lordosis influence sagittal cervical spine flexion extension kinematics in cervical spondylotic radiculopathy subjects? J Back Musculoskelet Rehabil. 2017, 30: 937-941.

[13] Moustafa IM, Diab AA, Taha S, Harrison DE. Addition of a Sagittal Cervical Posture Corrective Orthotic Device to a Multimodal Rehabilitation Program Improves Short- and Long-Term Outcomes in Patients with Discogenic Cervical Radiculopathy. Arch Phys Med Rehabil. 2016, 97: 2034-2044.

[14] Moustafa IM, Diab AA, Harrison DE. Does improvement towards a normal cervical sagittal configuration aid in the management of lumbosacral radiculopathy: A randomized controlled trial Proceedings of the 13th World Federation of Chiropractic Biennial Congress / ECU Convention, Athens, Greece, May 13-16, 2015. Paper #184 Mediterranean Region Award Winning Paper.

[15] Moustafa IM, Diab AA. Extension traction treatment for patients with discogenic lumbosacral radiculopathy: a randomized controlled trial. Clin Rehabil. 2012; Jan;27(1):51-62.

[16] Moustafa IM, Diab AM, Ahmed A, Harrison DE. The efficacy of cervical lordosis rehabilitation for nerve root function, pain, and segmental motion in cervical spondylotic radiculopathy. PhysioTherapy 2011; 97 Supplement: 846-847.

[17] Berry RH, Oakley PA, Harrison DE. Is one cause of trigeminal neuralgia subluxation of craniocervical posture? A CBP® case report. J Contemporary Chiro. 2020;3:28-35.

[18] Haas JW, Oakley PA, Harrison DE. Cervical pseudo-scoliosis reduction and alleviation of dystonia symptoms using Chiropractic BioPhysics® (CBP®) technique: A case report with a 1.5-year follow-up. J Contemp Chiropr. 2019; 2:131-137.

[19] Anderson JM, Oakley PA, Harrison DE. Improving posture to reduce the symptoms of Parkinson's: a CBP® case report with a 21 month follow-up. J Phys Ther Sci. 2019 Feb;31(2):153-158.

[20] Breton PY, Oakley PA, Harrison DE. Complete resolution of carpal tunnel syndrome after relieving the 'first crush' in 'double crush syndrome' by improving the cervical spine posture: A CBP® case report. J Contemp Chiropr. 2018; 2:49-53.

[21] Oakley PA, Harrison DE, Haas JW, Listenmaa SK. Positive Outcome with Tourette Syndrome and Chronic Tic Disorder Following Chiropractic Intervention: a Chiropractic Biophysics® (CBP) Case Report with a 13-year follow-up. Chiropr J Australia. 2017; 45(4):368-376.

[22] Oakley P, Harrison D. Restoration of barefoot gait in a 75-year old female with cervical spondylotic myelopathy: A case report utilizing Chiropractic BioPhysics (CBP®) technique. Chiropr J Australia. 2017; 45(1):16-27.

[23] Berry RH, Oakley P, Harrison D. Alleviation of radiculopathy by structural rehabilitation of the cervical spine by correcting a lateral head translation posture (-TxH) using Berry translation traction as a part of CBP methods: A case report. Chiropr J Australia. 2017; 45(1):63-72.

[24] Wickstrom BM, Oakley PA, Harrison DE. Non-surgical relief of cervical radiculopathy through reduction of forward head posture and restoration of cervical lordosis: a case report. J Phys Ther Sci. 2017 Aug;29(8):1472-1474.

[25] Oakley PA, Harrison DE. Lumbar extension traction alleviates symptoms and facilitates healing of disc herniation/sequestration in 6-weeks, following failed treatment from three previous chiropractors: a CBP® case report with an 8 year follow-up. J Phys Ther Sci. 2017 Nov;29(11):2051-2057.

[26] Breig A. Skull traction and spinal cord injury. A new approach to improved rehabilitation. New York, Springer-Verlag. 1989.

[27] Artz NJ, Adams MA, Dolan P. Sensorimotor function of the cervical spine in healthy volunteers. Clin Biomech. 2015;30: 260-268.

[28] Treleaven J. Sensorimotor disturbances in neck disorders affecting postural stability, head and eye movement control. Man Ther. 2008; 13: 2-11.

[29] Riemann BL, Lephart SM. The Sensorimotor System, Part II: The Role of Proprioception in Motor Control and Functional Joint Stability. J Athl Train. 2002; 37: 80-84.

[30] Hellström F, Roatta S, Thunberg J, Passatore M, Djupsjöbacka M. Responses of muscle spindles in feline dorsal neck muscles to electrical stimulation of the cervical sympathetic nerve. Exp brain Res. 2005; 165: 328-342.

[31] Corneil BD, Olivier E, Munoz DP. Neck Muscle Responses to Stimulation of Monkey Superior Colliculus. II. Gaze Shift Initiation and Volitional Head Movements. J Neurophysiol. 2002; 88: 2000-2018.

[32] Bolton PS, Kerman IA, Woodring SF, Yates BJ. Influences of neck afferents on sympathetic and respiratory nerve activity. Brain Res Bull. 1998; 47: 413-419.

[33] Budgell BS. Reflex effects of subluxation: the autonomic nervous system. J Manipulative Physiol Ther. 2000; 23: 104-106.

[34] Moustafa IM, Youssef A, Ahbouch A, Tamim M, Harrison DE. Is forward head posture relevant to autonomic nervous system function and cervical sensorimotor control? Cross sectional study. Gait Posture. 2020; 77:29-35.

[35] Oakley PA, Moustafa IM, Harrison DE. Restoration of cervical and lumbar lordosis: CBP® methods overview. In: Bettany-Saltikov J. Spinal Deformities in Adolescents, Adults and Older Adults. IntechOpen Publishers. 2020; Pp.1-19.

[36] Harrison DD, Janik TJ, Harrison GR, et al. Chiropractic biophysics technique: a linear algebra approach to posture in chiropractic. J Manipulative Physiol Ther. 1996, 19: 525-535.

[37] Oakley PA, Harrison DD, Harrison DE, Haas JW. Evidence-based protocol for structural rehabilitation of the spine and posture: review of clinical biomechanics of posture (CBP) publications. J Can Chiropr Assoc. 2005; 49(4):270-296.

[38] Harrison DE, Harrison DD, Hass JW. Structural rehabilitation of the cervical spine. Evanston, WY: Harrison CBP® Seminars, Inc., 2002.

[39] Harrison DE, Betz JW, Harrison DD, et al. CBP structural rehabilitation of the lumbar spine: Harrison Chiropractic Biophysics Seminars, 2007.

[40] Harrison DD, Janik TJ, Troyanovich SJ, Holland B. Comparisons of Lordotic Cervical Spine Curvatures to a Theoretical Ideal Model of the Static Sagittal Cervical Spine. Spine. 1996;21(6):667-675.

[41] Harrison DD, Janik TJ, Troyanovich SJ, Harrison DE, Colloca CJ. Evaluations of the Assumptions Used to Derive an Ideal Normal Cervical Spine Model. J Manipulative Physiol Ther. 1997;20(4):246-256.

[42] Harrison DD, Harrison DE, Janik TJ, Cailliet R, Haas JW, Ferrantelli J, Holland B. Modeling of the Sagittal Cervical Spine as a Method to Discriminate Hypo-Lordosis: Results of Elliptical and Circular Modeling in 72 Asymptomatic Subjects, 52 Acute Neck Pain Subjects, and 70 Chronic Neck Pain Subjects. Spine. 2004;29:2485-2492.

[43] Harrison DE, Janik TJ, Harrison DD, Cailliet R, Harmon S. Can the thoracic kyphosis be modeled with a simple geometric shape? The results of circular and elliptical modeling in 80 asymptomatic subjects. J Spinal Disord. 2002;15(3):213-220.

[44] Harrison DE, Harrison DD, Janik TJ, Cailliet R, Haas JW. Do alterations in vertebral and disc dimensions affect an elliptical model of the thoracic kyphosis? Spine. 2003;28(5):463-469.

[45] Troyanovich SJ, Cailliet R, Janik TJ, Harrison DD, Harrison DE. Radiographic mensuration characteristics of the sagittal lumbar spine from a normal population with a method to synthesize prior studies of lordosis. J Spinal Disord. 1997;10(5):380-386.

[46] Janik TJ, Harrison DD, Cailliet R, Troyanovich SJ, Harrison DE. Can the Sagittal Lumbar Curvature be Closely Approximated by an Ellipse? J Orthop Res. 1998;16(6):766-770.

[47] Harrison DD, Cailliet R, Janik TJ, Troyanovich SJ, Harrison DE, Holland B. Elliptical Modeling of the Sagittal Lumbar Lordosis and Segmental Rotation Angles as a Method to Discriminate Between Normal and Low Back Pain Subjects. J Spinal Disord. 1998;11(5):430-439.

[48] Harrison DE, Harrison DD, Cailliet R, Troyanovich SJ, Janik TJ, Holland B. Cobb method or Harrison posterior tangent method: which to choose for lateral cervical radiographic analysis. Spine. 2000;25(16):2072-2078.

[49] Harrison DE, Cailliet R, Harrison DD, Janik TJ, Holland B. Centroid, Cobb or Harrison posterior tangents: which to choose for analysis of thoracic kyphosis? Spine. 2001;26(11): E227-E234.

[50] Harrison DE, Cailliet R, Harrison DD, Janik TJ, Holland B. Radiographic analysis of lumbar lordosis: Cobb method, centroidal method, TRALL or Harrison posterior tangents? Spine. 2001;26(11):E235-E242.

[51] Harrison DE, Holland B, Harrison DD, Janik TJ. Further reliability analysis of the Harrison radiographic line drawing methods: Crossed ICCs for lateral posterior tangents and AP Modified-Riser Ferguson. J Manipulative Physiol Ther. 2002;25:93-98.

[52] Harrison DE, Harrison DD, Colloca CJ, et al. Repeatability over time of posture, radiograph positioning, and radiograph line drawing: An analysis of six control groups. J Manipulative Physiol Ther. 2003;26:87-98.

[53] McAviney J, Schulz D, Bock R, Harrison DE, Holland B. Determining the relationship between cervical lordosis and neck complaints. J Manipulative Physiol Ther. 2005;28(3):187-193.

[54] Harrison DD, Jackson BL, Troyanovich S, Robertson G, de George D, Barker WF. The efficacy of cervical extension-compression traction combined with diversified manipulation and drop table adjustments in the rehabilitation of cervical lordosis: a pilot study. J Manipulative Physiol Ther. 1994;17(7):454-464.

[55] Harrison DE, Harrison DD, Cailliet R, Janik TJ, Holland B. Changes in sagittal lumbar configuration with a new method of extension traction: non-randomized clinical control trial. Arch Phys Med Rehab. 2002;83(11):1585-1591.

[56] Harrison DE, Cailliet R, Harrison DD, Janik TJ, Holland B. New 3-Point bending traction method of restoring cervical lordosis combined with cervical manipulation: non-randomized clinical control trial. Arch Phys Med Rehab. 2002;83(4):447-453.

[57] Harrison DE, Harrison DD, Betz J, Colloca CJ, Janik TJ, Holland B. Increasing the cervical lordosis with seated combined extension-compression and transverse load cervical traction with cervical manipulation: non-randomized clinical control trial. J Manipulative Physiol Ther. 2003;26(3):139-151.

[58] Harrison DE, Harrison DD, Haas JW, Betz JW, Janik TJ, Holland B. Conservative methods to correct lateral translations of the head: a non-randomized clinical control trial. J Rehab Res Devel. 2004;41(4):631-640.

[59] Harrison DE, Cailliet R, Betz JW, Harrison DD, Haas JW, Janik TJ, Holland B. Harrison mirror image methods for correcting trunk list: a non-randomized clinical control trial. Eur Spine J. 2005;14(2):155-162.

[60] Diab AA, Moustafa IM. Rehabilitation for pain and lumbar segmental motion in chronic mechanical low back pain: a randomized trial. J Manipulative Physiol Ther. 2012;35(4):246-253.

[61] Diab AA, Moustafa IM. The efficacy of lumbar extension traction for sagittal alignment in mechanical low back pain. a randomized trial. J Back Musculoskelet Rehabil. 2013;26(2):213-222.

[62] Moustafa IM. Does improvement towards a normal cervical configuration aid in the management of fibromyalgia. A randomized controlled trial. Bull Fac Phys Ther Cairo Univ. 2013;18(2):29-41.

[63] Moustafa IM, Diab AA, Hegazy F, Harrison DE. Does improvement towards a normal cervical sagittal configuration aid in the management of cervical myofascial pain syndrome: a 1- year randomized controlled trial. BMC Musculoskelet Disord. 2018;19(1):396.

[64] Moustafa IM, Diab AA, Harrison DE. The Effect of Normalizing the Sagittal Cervical Configuration for the Management of Cervicogenic Headaches: A 2-Year Pilot Randomized Controlled Trial. J Rehabilitation Med. 2021; In Press.

[65] Lee SH, Kim KT, Seo EM, Suk KS, Kwack YH, Son ES. The influence of thoracic inlet alignment on the craniocervical sagittal balance in asymptomatic adults. J Spinal Disord Tech. 2011;25(2):E41–E47.

[66] Vrtovec T, Janssen MM, Likar B, Castelein RM, Viergever MA, Pernuš F. Evaluation of pelvic morphology in the sagittal plane. Spine J. 2013;13(11):1500-1509.

[67] Panjabi MM, White III AA. Biomechanics in the musculoskeletal system. New York: Churchill Livingstone, 2001.

[68] McCormick PC, Stein BM. Functional anatomy of the spinal cord and related structures. Neurosurgery Clinics of North America. 1990;1:469-489.

[69] Panjabi MM, White III AA. Biomechanics of nonacute cervical spinal cord trauma. Spine. 1988;13:838-842.

[70] Raynor RB, Koplik B. Cervical cord trauma. the relationship between clinical symptoms and force of injury. Spine. 1985;10:193-197.

[71] Breig A. Overstretching of and circumscribed pathological tension in the spinal cord: A basic cause of symptoms in cord disorders. J of Biomech. 1970;3:7-9.

[72] Stein JS. Failure of magnetic resonance imaging to reveal the cause of a progressive cervical myelopathy related to postoperative spinal deformity. Am J Phys Med Rehab. 1997;76:73-75.

[73] Breig A, Turnbull I, Hassler O. Effects of mechanical stresses on the spinal cord in cervical spondylosis: A study on fresh cadaver material. J Neurosurg. 1966;25:45-56.

[74] Harrison DE, Cailliet R, Harrison DD, Troyanovich SJ, Harrison SO. A review of biomechanics of the central nervous system Part II: Spinal cord strains from postural loads. J Manipulative Physiol Ther. 1999;22:322-332.

[75] Breig A, Marions O. Biomechanics of the lumbosacral nerve roots. Acta Radiologica Diagnosis 1963;1: 1141-1160.

[76] Jarzem PF, Quance DR, Doyle DJ, Begin LR, Kostuik JP. Spinal cord tissue pressure during spinal cord distraction in dogs. Spine. 1992 Aug;17(8 Suppl): S227–S234.

[77] Harrison DE, Cailliet R, Harrison DD, Troyanovich SJ, Harrison SO. A review of biomechanics of the central nervous system--Part III: spinal cord stresses from postural loads and their neurologic effects. J Manipulative Physiol Ther. 1999;22(6):399-410.

[78] Moustafa IM, Diab AAM, Taha S, Harrison DE. Demonstration of central conduction time and neuroplastic changes after cervical lordosis rehabilitation in asymptomatic subjects: A randomized, placebo-controlled trial. Proceedings of the 14th biennial congress of the World Federation of Chiropractic, March 15-18, 2017.

[79] Moustafa IM, Diab AA, Harrison DE: The effect of normalizing the sagittal cervical configuration on dizziness, neck pain, and cervicocephalic kinesthetic sensibility: a 1-year randomized controlled study. Eur J Phys Rehabil Med. 2017, 53: 57-71.

[80] Tousignant M, Duclos E, Laflèche S, Mayer A, Tousignant-Laflamme Y, Brosseau L, et al. Validity study for the cervical range of motion device used for lateral flexion in patients with neck pain. Spine. 2002; 27: 812-817.

[81] Testerman C, Vander Griend R. Evaluation of ankle instability using the Biodex Stability System. Foot Ankle Int. 1999;20:317-321.

[82] Schmitz R, Arnold B. Intertester and Intratester Reliability of a Dynamic Balance Protocol Using the Biodex Stability System, J Sport Rehabil. 1998; 7: 95-101.

[83] Tjell C, Rosenhall U. Smooth pursuit neck torsion test: a specific test for cervical dizziness. Am J Otol. 1998; 19: 76-81.

Section 3

Approaches Related to Specific Neurological Disorders

Chapter 5

Design of a Standing Device for Children with Spinal Dysraphysm

Aydeé Robayo-Torres and Katherine Quiñones-Argote

Abstract

The standing posture is one of the most important factors in the maturation of the neuromotor system, and it is an evolutionary necessity that phylogenetically makes possible the differentiation of functions between the upper and lower limbs, influencing a greater development of the latter; with a fundamental change in the shape of the foot: it increases the importance of the tarsus and metatarsus and reduces the work of the fingers, which facilitates the movement, transfer and independence of the individual in their activities of daily life. The design and production of the prototype of the device, the judgment of the experts, as well as the results of the physiotherapeutic evaluation before and after the standing program, are the threads that are woven in this research proposal. This study seeks to propose a prototype of a standing frame for pediatric patients with spina bifida. The design of a device for standing is proposed based on the individual characteristics of the users, which was evaluated by experts to later perform a case study on a standing program with this type of device in pediatric patients with spine bifida. The designed prototype seems to offer adequate conditions for maintaining standing and on some musculoskeletal conditions of the patient studied. The study concludes that assisted standing should be promoted through inexpensive, functional and continuous monitoring devices. A user-applied design is proposed and not a generic device model.

Keywords: standing, device, children, spinal dysraphysm, stander, Congenital abnormalities

1. Introduction

Children and adults who due to their motor disability situation, who cannot adopt the bipedal position, have a greater propensity to complications related to the decrease in bone mineral density, development of myo-tendon contractures, greater risk of gastrointestinal problems, less support of the diaphragm by the effect of gravity; increasing the risk of pressure ulcers because by not having the adequate redistribution of pressure in the ischial tuberosity, sacrum, spinous processes, scapulae and other bony prominences, blood perfusion that the tissues need is not allowed, thus increasing the risk of rupture of the skin in a seated individual. In addition, the possibility of presenting problems in the functioning of the bladder and greater predisposition to urinary tract infections [1].

One of the causes of disability is neural tube defects, which are the most serious congenital malformations of the central nervous system and the spine. They are the second major congenital anomaly after cardiac malformations, with a frequency that ranges between 0.5 and 2 per 1000 pregnancies, although in some geographical regions, for example, in northern China, frequencies of up to 10 per 1000 births. Furthermore, they account for up to 29% of neonatal deaths associated with congenital anomalies in low-income settings. Both the clinical manifestations and the resulting disabilities and mortality depend on its level and extent [2]. The structural defect occurs at any level of the neuraxis, from the brain to the sacrum; These neural tube defects located in the spine are classified as occult spina bifida and open or cystic spina bifida, in the latter, spina bifida is present, but accompanied by a protrusion of a meningeal sac with cerebrospinal fluid with neural tissue inside or without it and are classified as Meningocele, Myelomeningocele and Rachischisis with Mieloschisis. Myelomeningocele is the most serious form of spina bifida cystica that presents as a chronic disease, it produces a strong psychosocial impact on the child and their family since the child may present motor, urological, orthopedic and sometimes cognitive impairment [3, 4]. This can be done damaging effects on a child's well-being, education, and social engagement [5, 6].

Failure to adopt bipedal position implies the limitation of voluntary motor skills such as locomotion, transfers and self-care, sphincter involvement, restricting social and school participation. This is the reason why orthotic attachments or devices to achieve the maintenance of the bipedal position, have been proposed since time immemorial [7].

Recent research even recommends a "24-hour postural management program that you should consider including both a passive standing component and an active component using a stander that steps, vibrates, oscillates, sways, turns, bounces, moves from sit-to-stand under users' own power, allows users to self-propel, and so on, or other devices that combine weight-bearing and movement such as a gait trainer/support walker" [8].

Assisted standing involves using a device to help place load through a person's feet. Standing devices and orthoses provide a stable mechanical support for weight bearing in the supine, prone or upright positions, depending on the device chosen; however, a precise and timely evaluation of individual needs must select the most appropriate design of standing device, orthoses, or both. These benefits include preservation of muscle length and range of joint movement via the stretch that occurs during standing (predominantly of the hip and lower-limb muscles), delayed onset of scoliosis, increased bone density (thereby reducing the risk of fractures), fewer muscle spasms and better respiratory function (including voice control). Research on standing for other conditions has also suggested improved circulation, digestion, and bowel and bladder function. Clinical opinion on standing indicates other benefits, including pressure relief (which improves skin integrity), improvement of well-being and better sleep [9, 10].

In addition, for these people, there is the social stigma of depending on others for functional mobility, which is why an assistive device is necessary that facilitates the bipedal position, ambulation in the environment and development of activities typical of age, without assistance from another person and who contribute positively to society as a whole [11, 12].

One of the fields of the human body movement professional is precisely the design, prescription and evaluation of the use of this type of device for standing, known as Standing Stands. However, the limited and timid research that researchers have found in this field is surprising [13].

2. Material and methods

The approach to the design of machinery that was proposed in this project considered for its realization the steps of the engineering design flow [14], that is to say:

1. Recognition of a need.

2. Specifications and requirements that the machine must meet to solve the need.

3. Study of the possibilities.

   The purpose of the probability study is to verify the possible success or failure of a proposal, both from a technical and economic perspective.

4. Synthesis of creative design.

   In this phase of design, researchers must act as physiotherapists, "empirical engineers," inventors, and artists, to create the machine.

5. Preliminary design and development.

   Drawings of the machine as a whole and of the specific parts of it, the dimensions and important notations, as well as auxiliary sectional views, that fully explain the proposed design. In addition, kinematic studies are conducted, which include the design of the machine and the possible movements that it should conduct.

6. Detailed design.

   Detailed design refers to the actual rigging and sizing of all individual components, both purchased and manufactured, that make up the total product, device, or system. The assistance of experts in the different areas was necessary in order to carry out the stander on the right track.

7. Prototype construction and testing.

   At this stage, the parts were manufactured, the commercial components were purchased and the machine or system, after the assembly, is ready for evaluation and testing. After the necessary changes and/or modifications have been made, the new components are incorporated into the prototype assembly to continue with the tests and evaluations. This process was performed until the designer, in this case the researchers, were satisfied with the stipulated specifications.

8. Production design, this stage is not part of this project as it is a pilot test.

   This was the prototype of the standing frame that was used in the case, which was subjected to evaluation in the prototype workshop of the Faculty of Engineering of the National University, and to an expert judgment (**Figure 1**).

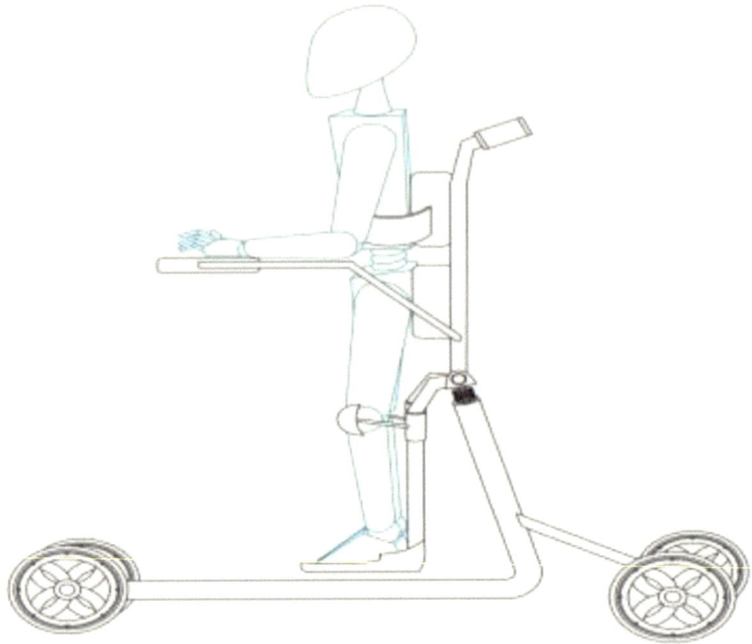

Figure 1.
Graphic design of the prototype.

Based on the prototype, a case study was designed with a 10-year-old patient with myelomeningocele type spina bifida level T12 - L4, the most relevant sequelae of which were bilateral-grade IV/V vesicourethral reflux, flaccid neurogenic bladder in catheterization intermittent from the age of 4 years old, bilateral hydronephrosis, bilateral dysplasia of the hips and coxa varas, flaccid paraplegia, among others.

The researchers understood, assumed and classified this research project as minimal risk, given that other stanchions have been created in the world, which have facilitated the study and description of the risks derived from its use in the adult population [15], and to a lesser extent in the pediatric population, with an inability to acquire the bipedal position. The possible risks, their handling and control are known and foreseen by the researchers. These risks include signs of orthostatism, diaphoresis, emesis, pressure zones, allergy to materials, tinnitus, paresthesia, fall, tachycardia, bradypnea or polypnea [16].

The benefit derived from the use of the stander was based on the care of the conditions that generally affect people unable to adopt the bipedal position [1]. Therefore, in the cost–benefit ratio, the risks inherent to the research were widely outweighed by the benefits provided by assisted standing in this type of population, being a novel and reasonable orthosis, insofar as it was intended to attend a sequel and a need that the Colombian health system is not prepared to meet and has completely neglected in the research study subject.

Confidentiality was guaranteed by the researchers for both the study subject and his family.

According to Title III of the current regulations, in this study an informed consent was obtained for the research subject, with prior evaluation by the psychology service of the Faculty of Medicine of the National University in which it was certified that the subject of study, can understand, reason and logic, which allows you to understand the importance and role of your participation in this research. In the same way, they proceeded to obtain informed consent from their parents.

3. Results from the expert judgment

A search was carried out for experts in various areas such as pediatric neurology, biomedical engineering, biomechanics and medical technology; who could evaluate the different characteristics of the stander. For this, five expert professionals were contacted, of which 80% were physiotherapists and 20% belonged to mechanical engineering.

4. Criteria for the evaluation of the stander

The characteristics of both the shape (design, safety, resistance, weight, mobility, esthetics, among others) and the bottom of the standing frame were evaluated with a view to incorporate the changes, modifications and suggestions received by the judges into the final prototype. At the request of one of the evaluators, the researchers made a technical specification sheet, which could unify a technical language that is understandable to the reader. The evaluation was conducted using the following qualification criteria:

1. Excellent

2. Very good

3. Good

4. Regular

5. Bad

6. Very bad

4.1 Design creativity

The grade point average for this criterion was excellent.

One aspect highlighted by one of the experts was the fact of considering standard measures of Colombian architecture, such as the width of the doors, and the standardized measures of wheelchairs, to provide better accessibility to various spaces.

4.2 Security provided by the patient standard

In this criterion, the experts argued that some improvements must increase safety, such as lateral supports on the back and seat. Another evaluator expressed concern about how safe an obese patient might be. The average grade for this criterion was very good.

4.3 Design of supports to avoid pressure zones in the body segments

The average qualification for this criterion was very good, although we insist on reviewing any pressure zones.

4.4 Materials used for creation the stander

The testers expressed that they look tough and that they are suitable for durability and strength. Another evaluator requested a technical sheet of the stander and the value of the resistance of the materials. The grade point average for this criterion was very good. One of the elements highlighted in the structure was the use of a special weld, which guarantee safety in the different joints of the standing frame.

4.5 Structural strength of the staircase

In this item, the evaluators stated that the design and manufacture guaranties the resistance of the stanchion and suggested performing load-bearing tests for a more generalized use. The grade point average for this criterion was very good.

Considering that the structural resistance of the prototype is fundamental, the researchers consulted with a mechanical engineer to make a 3D modeling, in which a simulation was intended to find resistance values and critical points in the structure. Regarding the load-bearing test, when manufacturing the prototype, a static test with a weight of 100 kg was performed for 24 hours, finding that the structures did not suffer any damage. However, to conduct other types of tests, it must have another manufactured stanchion, which is available only to measure with what applied force it could suffer some damage.

4.6 Weight of the staircase

The evaluators stated that it is a bit heavy, however it is much lighter than other types of stanchions that do not have an electric motorization system; They also expressed that another type of material such as aluminum could reduce the weight. The grade point average for this criterion was very good.

4.7 Ease of handling

In this evaluation criterion, the evaluators stated that they are concerned about children with spina bifida who have attention and coordination difficulties, they stated that the regulatory system could be improved to make it easier for the family to manipulate, modifying it to a system of pin commonly used on crutches and canes; it is also required to improve transportability. The grade point average for this criterion was very good.

4.8 Expansion capacity in the different segments whereas loads is produced

The experts expressed that the stander offers wide possibilities to adjust the size in different parts of it, although some adjustments are required to improve the expansion capacity in the seat. The grade point average for this criterion was excellent.

4.9 Stander dimensions

The experts stated that they were adequate to achieve difficult accesses, although, if it does not risk stability, it would be preferable to shorten it a bit; another expert said he finds it a bit cumbersome to fit into an average car. The rating for this criterion was very good.

4.10 Esthetic appearance in shape, textures, accessories, colors, among others

The evaluators stated that the colors were very striking, had very special details and colors with a specific objective. The grade point average for this criterion was very good.

4.11 Ease off cleaning the staircase

The stander met the hygiene requirements set by the researchers and evaluators. The grade point average for this criterion was very good.

4.12 What other evaluation item would you formulate?

The experts proposed the following form evaluation criteria for the stander:

- Durability of materials
- Inquire about costs
- Manipulation by the family

In the same way, the group of experts made the following contributions from the open questions:

- Check the push bar, as safety concerns for the people accompanying the child, their companions or caregivers. Regarding this recommendation, the researchers proceeded to shorten the bar by 30 cm, to avoid accidents in other people.
- Consider foot deformities, specifically the tendency to clubfoot, added to the absence or little sensitivity in relation to the footrest. Here, the patient has an AFO type orthosis, which favors the stabilization of these segments, even more so when acquiring the bipedal position. However, this aspect should be reviewed at the time of series production.
- Pelvic belt and foot safety at 45°, with Velcro: regarding the angulation of the pelvic belt, it would be necessary to do it in the case in which the prototype only offered the possibility of maintaining the sitting position, however, when also assisting the position bipedal, a position must be found that ensures stability in both positions.
- Abductor stop: the population with altered tone requires this help. This modification is intended to be conducted in subsequent prototypes.
- Wider wheels: for the rear wheels, it is possible to carry out this modification, however for the front wheel it would involve a considerable increase in friction, which would not allow the user to easily direct the movement of the stander, consequently a complete change in steering system.
- Modification of the command panel: one of the evaluators considers that it is necessary to change some buttons, so that they are easier for the user to understand. Regarding this, the researchers performed a previous test, with

a child of the same age and schooling as the study subject, finding that after a brief instruction, the child was able to maneuver the standing frame in all directions, so no this modification is considered necessary.

4.13 Results of the implementation of the bipedestation in the subject of study

Making the comparison between the physiotherapeutic evaluation before and after the standing protocol in the study subject, it was found that:

- In the cardiovascular and respiratory dimension it was found:
  - On the scale of perceived exertion (modified Borg), the study subject initially considered standing activity with a rating of hard; after finishing the sessions, the rating decreased to soft.
  - When performing the evaluation of ventilatory mechanics, it was found that there was an increase of 0.5 cm in the thoracic expansion of the study subject.
- Regarding the anthropometric characteristics, the following changes were found:
  - In the initial evaluation, the BMI was in the 65th percentile and in the final evaluation it was in the 30th percentile. Despite this decrease, the BMI was in the normal ranges.
  - Regarding the perimeters, an increase of 1.5 cm was found in shoulders and abdomen; at the hip 2 cm; 1.7 cm for the right upper thigh and 2.7 cm for the left and 0.5 cm for the leg. Likewise, there was a decrease in some perimeters, such as 1 cm in the right middle thigh and 0.8 cm in the lower thigh.
- In the positive internal contextual factors and participation, it was found that the patient improved her mood after the start of standing, has greater initiative to conduct different activities that she did not do before, such as helping to wash the dishes after eating, help serve in the store of their parents.
- Regarding integumentary and vascular integrity, it was found:
  - Regarding the pressure ulcer presented by the study subject, it was found that in the initial evaluation, it had dimensions of 2.4 cm wide x 1.5 cm high; in the final evaluation it was 2.1 cm wide x 1 cm high. This shows a decrease of 0.3 cm in width and 0.5 cm in height in the crater.
- Regarding joint integrity and mobility, the results obtained can be seen in **Table 1**:
- In the muscle evaluation, a slight contraction was found in the hip flexor muscles on both sides in the final evaluation.
- In the evaluation of sensory and neuromotor integrity it was found:
  - Superficial sensitivity: when evaluating touch and pain, it was obtained that the study subject initially reported perceiving the stimuli up to the level of T12 on the left side and T11 on the right side. In the final evaluation, a

Joint	Range of motion
Gain	
Right and left hip flexion	22°
Right hip internal rotation	26°
Left hip internal rotation	16°
Left hip external rotation	7°
Left knee flexion	6°
Knee extension	10°
Right foot neck inversion	5°
Left foot neck inversion	3°
Right foot neck eversion	30°
Left foot neck eversion	25°
Decrease	
Hip adduction	17°
Left foot neck dorsiflexion	15°
Right metatarsophalangeal flexion	18°
Left metatarsophalangeal flexion	30°
Bilateral metatarsophalangeal extension	10°

Table 1.
Comparison of gain and decrease in the ranges of motion obtained in the pre and post physiotherapeutic evaluations.

perception of the stimulation was obtained on the lateral aspect of L2 in the right hemibody and up to L1 in the left side.

- ASIA: in the initial evaluation, the sensitive level was T11 and in the final evaluation it was L1. The motor level remained the same in the two evaluations, however in the final evaluation a slight contraction of the hip flexors was found.

- In the postural analysis the following results were found:
  - Postural alignment in sitting position: pelvic obliquity changed the score from slight elevation of 10° to the right side to normal; the lateral displacement of the trunk was maintained in a grade of mild, going from a displacement of 5° to the left to a 5° displacement to the right; lateral head tilt changed from Tilt 10° to the right (slight) to normal; hip rotation remained normal in both evaluations; posterior pelvic tilt, thoracic and lumbar curvature remained the same in the two evaluations; in the posterior inclination of the head there was a decrease of 13°, going from slight to normal; slight pelvic rotation remained the same in both evaluations; in the adduction and abduction of the hips a grade of normal was maintained.
  - Positive Galeazzi sign, finding a decrease in the difference of 0.9 cm, with the lower right limb is the lowered one.
  - Spine: mobility was evaluated with the Schober test, finding an increase of 1 cm in the displacement of the vertebrae. The alignment of the spine was also

evaluated with the Adams test, which shows an increase in curvature toward the left side in the dorsal area, maintaining the same result in both evaluations.

The researchers also consider it pertinent mentioning other changes that occurred in the study subject during assisted standing; These data were obtained from the parents' narratives during the course of the investigation and will be presented below:

- In relation to the musculoskeletal system, the parents report that "when palpating the muscles of the thighs and legs of the study subject, they found a considerable increase in their hardness (muscular turgor)."

- In relation to the stability and postsurgical ossification of the pelvis and hip, radiographic images are obtained after the process of standing, whose examinations are in the hands of the parents and which, according to them, in an appointment made with orthopedics, the doctor The practitioner noted a rare improvement in the stability and ossification of the pelvis and hip.

- Regarding urine color, appearance and volume, the parents decreased the consumption of this drug in the study subject, even stopping the use of this antibiotic during standing.

- In the digestive system, the parents reported that from the second week of assisted standing, the fecal bolus changed its appearance, going from hard goat-type stools to soft stools that looked more like normal. Parents mentioned that this event had never been presented; It is also important to mention that the use of the medicated laxative (PEG) were suspended due to the positive change in the consistency of the stool.

- Regarding the participation of the individual, a favorable change was achieved in the emotional part of the study subject, a better disposition was also generated to perform activities in which they did not usually participate, such as cleaning the home, helping their parents with work typical of home and work.

- Regarding the movement of the subject, the parents report an improvement in stability, alignment of the trunk and lower limbs, and the ease with which they crawl inside the home.

According to these results, it is observed that it is necessary to design these devices based on the individual characteristics of each patient/user, so as to guarantee an adequate man–machine correlation and therefore obtain better results derived from the use of the device. This is why this research bets on a personalized design and not in series, economic, light and esthetic, unlike most of the stanchions.

The researchers recognize the importance of having received training in various areas that contributed to the development of the research, however, a limitation of the study corresponds to a gap in training in terms of basic elements of design and production of orthotic devices or attachments and the review of other systems, such as bladder and gastrointestinal function, which are also a fundamental part of the human body movement, but which still do not have a concrete argument from the point of view of the physiotherapist. Therefore researchers would hope that a project will be proposed, hopefully in the short term, where this area is deepened and subjects are offered, where these issues and views are explored and reflected by physiotherapists in training.

5. Conclusions

After completing this investigative process, the researchers have reached the following conclusions:

- The intervention of the physiotherapists in terms of design and generation of structures and technologies that facilitate the habilitation and rehabilitation of the patient, from the paradigm of design applied to the user, are one of the intervention modalities that is most respectful of individual characteristics and context in which the orthosis is going to be implemented, so in the mediation between the human and the technological, a judicious monitoring of the process is necessary.

- The experiences reported by the experts show us that with the prototype produced in this research it is necessary and useful, while without neglecting its esthetic appearance, greater functionality was always sought in the patient.

- Assisted standing should be a right for the population with spina bifida, since kidney, gastrointestinal and respiratory diseases are the main reasons why these patients have a high level of morbidity and mortality. Therefore, devices such as the one proposed in this work, made with national materials and with Colombian design, 10 times cheaper than those on the market, could respond to these needs.

Author details

Aydeé Robayo-Torres[1*] and Katherine Quiñones-Argote[2]

1 Departamento del Movimiento Corporal Humano, Facultad de Medicina, Universidad Nacional de Colombia, Bogotá, Colombia

2 Universidad Nacional de Colombia, Bogotá, Colombia

*Address all correspondence to: alrobayot@unal.edu.co

References

[1] Meyer, A. (2008). For the benefits offered by standing, there are no alternatives. *The Interdisciplinary Journal of Rehabilitation.*

[2] Flores, S. (2019). Defectos del Tubo Neural: Factores de Riesgo Etiologico. *Rev Clin Esc Med*, 9(1), 65-71.

[3] Cruz, S., Bencomo, G., & Valladares, B. (2019). Congenital malformation of Spine, Myelomeningocele. Case report. *Rev Cub de Tec de la Sal*, 10(2),133-141.

[4] Aguirre, C., (2020). *Atención fisioterapéutica en paciente con espina bífida en la comunidad del valle del Chota de la provincia de Imbabura.* [Tesis, Universidad Tecnica del Norte]. Repositorio Institucional Universidad Tecnica del Norte. http://repositorio.utn.edu.ec/handle/123456789/10319

[5] Buckley BS, Sanders CD, Spineli L, Deng Q, Kwong JS. (2019). Conservative interventions for treating functional daytime urinary incontinence in children. *Cochrane Database Syst Rev*, 9(9), CD012367. doi: 10.1002/14651858.CD012367.pub2.

[6] Ramon, S. (2005). *El niño con espina bífida y su familia: el reto para el cuidado de enfermería.* [Monografia, Universidad de Antioquia]. Repositorio Institucional Universidad de Antioquia. http://bibliotecadigital.udea.edu.co/bitstream/10495/164/1/RamonSandra_2005_NinoEspinaBifida.pdf

[7] Serrano, M. (2008). Reacciones primitivas y reacciones neuromotoras: sustrato neurologico del comportamiento motor en el ser humano. *Revista Movimiento Científico*, 2(1), 3-4. https://revmovimiento cientifico.ibero.edu.co/article/view/308/276

[8] Paleg, G., Smith, B., & Glickman, L. (2013). Systematic review and evidence-based clinical recommendations for dosing of pediatric supported standing programs. *Pediatric Physical Therapy*, 25(3), 232-247.

[9] Pedlow, K., McDonough, S., Lennon, S., Kerr, C., & Bradbury, I. (2019). Assisted standing for Duchenne muscular dystrophy. *Cochrane Database Syst Rev*, 10(10), CD011550. doi: 10.1002/14651858.CD011550.pub2.

[10] Schmidt, C., Kaferle, J., Rydh, B. , Ahlborg, L., Hansen, H., Skjellvik, U., Thon, T., Damkjar, R., Pekanovic, A., Tornberg, A., & Lauruschkus, K. (2019). Effect of assisted walking-movement in patients with genetic and acquired neuromuscular disorders with the motorised Innowalk device: an international case study meta-analysis. *PeerJ, 7,* 70-98. https://doi.org/10.7717/peerj.7098

[11] Fenton, B. (2007). Standers can provide clients with both improved physical well-being and psychological benefits. *The Interdisciplinary Journal of Rehabilitation*.

[12] Valdivielso, A., & Mingo, M. (2019). *Abordaje fisioterapéutico de la marcha en pacientes pediátricos con espina bífida. Revisión bibliográfica*. [Tesis, Universidad de Valladolid]. Repositorio Institucional Universidad de Valladolid. http://uvadoc.uva.es/handle/10324/38775

[13] Niazi, Z., Salzberg, C., Byrne, D., & Viehbeck, M. (1997). Recurrence of initial pressure ulcer in persons with spinal cord injuries. *Adv Wound Care*, 10(3), 38-42.

[14] Lincoln, J. (1978). *Principles of Industrial Welding.* James F. Lincoln Arc Welding Foundation.

[15] Paleg, G. (2008). Synthesized literature review, Suported Standing. 3-13.

[16] Walker, C. (2013). *Fisioterapia en Obstetricia y Uroginecologia*. Elsevier Masson

Chapter 6

Dysphagia Associated with Neurological Disorders

Vadim I. Ershov

Abstract

Neurogenic dysphagia is characterized by problems with neural control of swallowing caused by various neurological diseases: vascular diseases, traumatic diseases, neoplasms, infections, neuromuscular diseases, and others. In patients of intensive care units after long-term intubation and extubation may evolve "postextubation dysphagia", characterized by the "learned non-use" phenomenon. Neurogenic dysphagia is a component of bulbar or pseudobulbar palsy, depending on the level of the neurological lesion. Diagnoses of neurogenic dysphagia include clinical examination (water swallow test), videofluoroscopy, upper gastrointestinal tract endoscopy and manometry, fiberoptic endoscopic evaluation of swallowing, a grade of Penetration-Aspiration Scale, and Fiberoptic Endoscopic Dysphagia Severity Scale. Dysphagia complications (malnutrition, dehydration, weight loss, aspiration, and respiratory tract obstruction) associated with bad functional recovery and life prognosis, so neurogenic dysphagia need a complex treatment: correct feeding pattern of caloric value and consistency, methods of oral cavity mucosa sensitivity stimulation, swallowing process stimulation, physiotherapeutic treatment methods (electrical stimulation of the larynx and tongue root), logopedic exercises therapy, surgical correction, lifestyle correction, and others. Sometimes it is a need for replacement therapy method by nasogastric tube and percutaneous endoscopic gastrostomy, parenteral feeding in several cases. Neurogenic dysphagia patient rehabilitation includes the "swallowing enhancement" method with optimal food consistency and training method after correct preparation of the oral cavity for swallowing. Neurogenic dysphagia patient oral feeding requires correct technique and contact with the patient for safety and efficient recovery.

Keywords: swallowing, dysphagia, stroke, rehabilitation

1. Introduction

Dysphagia is difficulty swallowing. Dysphagia is common in patients with neurological disorders. It can result from damage to the central or peripheral nervous system, as well as muscle and neuromuscular junction disorders. Neurogenic dysphagia often leads to serious complications including pulmonary aspiration, dehydration, and malnutrition. Dysphagia negatively affects the course of the disease and its outcome. Ethinenias can usually be prevented if dysphagia is detected early and treated correctly. The most common cause of neurogenic dysphagia, however, is stroke [1].

2. Physiological aspects of the swallowing process

Swallowing is a sequence of coordinated voluntary and involuntary (reflex) movements that push contents of the oral cavity into the esophagus and the stomach. It is a complex process consisting of coordinated movements of the jaw, the soft palate, and the esophagus muscles. The process involves the olivary nuclei and the cerebral cortex [2]. A person swallows approximately 600 times per day. Nearly 200 times while eating, 50 times while sleeping, and 350 times in all other cases. In most cases, swallowing is performed unconsciously [3].

The process of swallowing can be divided into four phases: oral, oropharyngeal, pharyngeal, and esophagopharyngeal. During the first (oral) phase, food is delivered into the oral cavity. Food is chewed, it is moistened with saliva, and a food bolus is formed [3, 4].

During the second (oropharyngeal) phase, the food is accumulated at the back of the tongue, chewing is stopped, and the tongue lifts up and pushes the food bolus through the pharynx into the middle portion of the pharynx (oropharynx). At the same time, the longitudinal muscles of the tongue and the mylohyoid muscles contract and press down the tip, back, and root of the tongue sequentially to the hard palate. The tongue is pushed backwards. The soft palate lifts up as to close down the nasopharynx. The pharynx and the hyoid bone move forward and up. The epiglottis moves back and down as to close down the entrance to the trachea. Breathing stops. The pharynx contracts [5].

During the third (pharyngeal) phase, the food bolus moves down into the middle portion of the pharynx, where the middle pharyngeal constrictor and the inferior pharyngeal constrictor contract, ensuring the bolus is squeezed and pushed downwards. At the same time, the larynx and the hyoid bone lifts up, enabling faster food bolus passing through the middle portion of the pharynx to the inferior portion. At the moment of swallowing, the reflex response enables expansion of the esophageal entrance, and the pharyngeal constrictors push the food bolus through the pyriform sinuses into the esophagus [5, 6].

During the fourth (esophagopharyngeal) phase, the upper esophageal sphincter relaxes. The food bolus enters the esophagus. The esophagus contracts sequentially. The inferior esophageal sphincter opens. The food bolus enters the stomach [6].

The first phase is voluntary, while the others are involuntary. Cranial nerves IX, X, XI are involved at all stages of swallowing [7].

Dysphagia (from dys- + Greek "phagein" meaning to eat, to swallow) is a clinical symptom of swallowing dysfunction: difficulty or painful passage of a food bolus from the oral cavity to the stomach [8]. Dysphagia can occur both as an independent condition or as a part of complex syndrome. Thus, dysphagia is the most important element of a bulbar or pseudobulbar palsy. Dysphagia is a subjective perception of difficulty swallowing.

Swallowing disorders are signs of various diseases. It is one of the key problems in diffuse and focal brain injuries [9]. Dysphagia occurs in 27.2% of elderly, who can take care of themselves; in 47.4% of elderly patients in intensive care units; in 51% of persons needing assistance. Dysphagia develops in 13–57% of patients suffering from dementia, in 19–81% of patients with Parkinson's disease, in 44–60% of patients with neurodegenerative diseases. Neurogenic dysphagia occurs in 25–65% of patients after stroke, provided that mortality rates among tube-fed patients with post-stroke dysphagia vary from 20 to 24% [2, 10]. In 15–17% of cases, difficulty swallowing develops after posterior fossa brain tumor surgeries and represents one of dangerous postoperative complications. Nearly 60% of patients experience difficulty swallowing after extubation [11, 12].

Dysphagia has a negative impact on the quality of life. It leads to severe respiratory complications; it becomes the cause of dehydration, metabolic disorders, and cachexia. Dysphagia increases disability, significantly worsens prognosis, and complicates patient rehabilitation. Dysphagia is a significant risk factor for the development of aspiration pneumonia [13].

3. Dysphagia classification

Dysphagia is commonly divided into esophageal and oropharyngeal.

Based on the functional mechanisms of disease development, dysphagia is classified into:

- neurogenic (motor, high)
- organic or mechanical
- psychogenic

In addition, all types of dysphagia can be divided into:

- acute
- chronic

Based on the disease course, dysphagia can be:

- intermittent
- persistent
- progressive, with increasing clinical symptoms

4. Pathogenesis of neurogenic dysphagia

In most cases, neurogenic dysphagia is oropharyngeal [14]. Neurogenic dysphagia is characterized by problems with neural control of swallowing caused by various neurological diseases.

The most common cause of neurogenic dysphagia development is a stroke [9–10, 15, 16]. Dysphagia can also occur in case of traumatic brain injury, brain tumors, encephalitis, botulism, and rabies. This type of pathology is observed at late stages of Parkinson's disease, Alzheimer's disease, amyotrophic lateral sclerosis, other neurodegenerative diseases, severe myasthenia gravis, multiple sclerosis, Guillain–Barré syndrome, and other disorders.

On rare occasions, neurogenic dysphagia can be the sole manifestation. However, in most cases it is a component of bulbar or pseudobulbar palsy (**Tables 1** and **2**).

Bulbar palsy occurs in case of bilateral or unilateral injury of cranial nerve nuclei IX, X, and XII and their roots. Isolated nuclear palsy is not common due to close proximity of anatomical structures of the caudal part of the medulla. Bulbar palsy elements are also included in some alternating syndromes. By its nature, bulbar palsy is peripheral paralysis of the pharynx. In addition to dysphagia, bulbar palsy is

Bulbar dysfunctions	Sensitivity of pharyngeal mucosa	Swallowing function	Epiglottis position (evaluation of the epiglottic paresis grade)
Grade 1	Partially preserved	Preserved	Upper (normal)
Grade 2	Partially preserved	Partially impaired	Upper
Grade 3	Not observed	Impaired	Upper
Grade 4	Not observed	Grossly impaired	Medium
Grade 5	Not observed	Not observed	Lower (epiglottic paralysis)

Table 1.
Bulbar dysfunction scale.

Variant	Clinical profile
1st	Partially preserved sensitivity of the laryngeal mucosa and the epiglottic mobility; the swallowing function is preserved. On rare occasions, choking starts when liquid food is swallowed; patients do not require tube feeding.
2nd	Mild impairment of swallowing function with partially preserved sensitivity of the laryngeal mucosa; patients experience significant limitations. These patients can be fed by small portions (using a teaspoon) with food of cream, puree, and jelly-like consistency. When a patient has impaired critical judgment and weak ability to concentrate on performed actions, a need for tube feeding arises.
3rd	Severe impairment of laryngeal mucosa sensitivity and severe impairment of swallowing function, which require tube feeding. This variant is the most dangerous in terms of underestimation of case severity, because the epiglottis is in its upper position and it does not block breathing. Aspiration of the oropharynx contents into the trachea is common. Due to impairment of laryngeal and tracheal mucosa sensitivity and cough reflex suppression, aspiration is manifested at late stages in the form of respiratory failure and rapidly progressive pneumonia.
4th	Severe impairment of laryngeal mucosa sensitivity, severe impairment of swallowing function; the epiglottis is in its middle position and usually does not block breathing. In this variant, aspiration is manifested quite soon after failure of respiratory tract protection in the form of respiratory failure and grunting breathing.
5th	Severe impairment of laryngeal mucosa sensitivity, no swallowing function. The epiglottis rests at the inferior wall of the larynx, i.e., in its lower position. The glottis can be examined only using a fiberscope or via direct laryngoscopy (during intubation). Respiratory failure in such patients is usually manifested immediately after failure of respiratory tract protection (extubation) in the form of difficulty breathing.

Table 2.
Variants of bulbar dysfunctions (swallowing function).

characterized by dysarthria (speech disorder resulting from an injury of the nerves responsible for articulation), atrophy of the pharynx and tongue muscles, and aphonia. As a rule, breathing pattern disorders (aspiration syndrome, Lambert–Eaton myasthenic syndrome, respiratory failure) develop in critically ill patients suffering from bulbar palsy, which often leads to death [17]. This is caused by close proximity of the caudal group of cranial nerve nuclei to the respiratory and vasomotor centers [7].

Pseudobulbar palsy is a neurological syndrome caused by bilateral disturbance of the corticonuclear tracts. In contrast to bulbar palsy, pseudobulbar palsy is central paralysis of the pharynx. Pseudobulbar palsy is characterized by the same triad of symptoms as bulbar palsy: dysarthria, dysphonia, and dysphagia. However, in pseudobulbar palsy, swallowing disorders are less severe: there is no muscles atrophy, primitive oral reflexes are present, and pharyngeal reflex does not disappear. Pseudobulbar palsy is characterized by compulsive crying or laughing. Pseudobulbar palsy can be often combined with signs of central hemiparesis or tetraparesis, due to the pyramidal tracts involvement [6, 7, 18].

A special form of oropharyngeal dysphagia called "postextubation dysphagia" (PED) was first observed in 1991 during myography of oral cavities of extubated patients. PED is one of the signs of post-intensive care syndrome (PICS) [2, 19–21]. The pathogenesis of PED is characterized by the "learned non-used" phenomenon characterized by three-phase swallowing impairment associated with long-term intubation (>48 h) or due to the absence of subglottal pressure in case of a cannula bearing [17, 22].

5. Neurogenic dysphagia diagnoses and monitoring

Dysphagia assessment procedures are selected depending on patient characteristics, severity of swallowing disorder, and procedure availability. Patients with stroke shall be screened for dysphagia during the first 24 hours after the disease onset and before oral eating [9, 23].

Swallowing assessment protocol was developed by the American Speech–Language–Hearing Association (ASHA). The main tests for oropharyngeal dysphagia assessment are the following ones:

- Water swallow test (three-swallow test): inexpensive and potentially useful basic screening test together with the data obtained from medical history and physical examination. The test has prognostic sensitivity of >95% as applied to detection of dysphagia occurrence [24, 25].

- Videofluoroscopy ("modified barium swallow"), which is a gold standard for oropharyngeal dysphagia assessment. The swallowing process is video recorded during fluoroscopy. Monitoring of patient's swallowing motions is provided. This procedure can be beneficial in predicting the risk of aspiration pneumonia [26].

- Upper gastrointestinal tract endoscopy. Endoscopy is not a sensitive method for detection of impaired swallowing function and is not effective for aspiration detection. At the same time, this method is effective for dysphagia monitoring [27].

- Fiberoptic endoscopic evaluation of swallowing (FEES), which is a modified method that includes visual examination of the larynx and pharynx structures using flexible transnasal fiberoptic endoscope when a patient is eating or drinking. This method is the most commonly used in real clinical practice [28].

- Overall estimate of dysphagia severity is based on summing up PAS and FEDS grades (**Tables 3–5**) [15, 27].

- Automated impedance-manometry (AIM), which is combination of impedance-manometry and high-resolution manometry. This method provides valuable diagnostic information. These measurements represent reliable prognostic method of aspiration [10, 29].

- High-resolution pharyngoesophageal manometry, which is quantitative assessment of pressure and time of the pharynx contraction and time of upper esophagus relaxation. It can be used in combination with videofluoroscopy in order to gain better understanding of involved movements and pressure [30].

Grading	Description of respiratory tract, larynx, and trachea state
1	Food does not pass into the respiratory tract.
2	Food passes into the respiratory tract, staying above the vocal cords and it can be coughed out of the respiratory tract.
3	Food passes into the respiratory tract, staying above the vocal cords but it cannot leave the respiratory tract.
4	Food passes into the respiratory tract, touches the vocal cords, and is pushed out of the respiratory tract.
5	Food passes into the respiratory tract, touches the vocal cords but cannot be pushed out of the respiratory tract.
6	Food passes into the respiratory tract, it passes beneath the vocal cords and cannot be pushed out of the larynx or respiratory tract.
7	Food passes into the respiratory tract, it passes beneath the vocal cords and cannot be pushed out of the trachea despite the efforts.
8	Food passes into the respiratory tract, it passes beneath the vocal cords, but a patient is too weak to cough it up.

Table 3.
Penetration-aspiration scale (PAS) developed according to Rosenbek criteria.

	Main findings	Grade	Potential clinical consequences
Saliva	Penetration/aspiration	Grade 6	No oral eating, only tube feeding
Pudding	Penetration or aspiration without or insufficient protective reflex	Grade 5	Tube feeding
Pudding	Penetration/aspiration with sufficient protective reflex	Grade 4	Tube feeding with small portions of pudding for oral eating during rehabilitation procedures
Liquids	Penetration or aspiration without or insufficient protective reflex	Grade 4	Tube feeding with small portions of pudding for oral eating during rehabilitation procedures
Liquids	Penetration/aspiration with sufficient protective reflex	Grade 3	Oral eating of pureed food
Solid food	Penetration/aspiration with food residues in the pyriform sinuses	Grade 2	Oral eating of pudding or liquids
Solid food	No penetration or aspiration, mild residues of food in the sinuses	Grade 1	Oral eating of semi-solid food or liquids

Table 4.
Fiberoptic endoscopic dysphagia severity scale (FEDSS).

Overall estimate	0 = no dysphagia	1 = mild dysphagia	2 = moderate dysphagia		3 = severe dysphagia		4 = very severe dysphagia	
Penetration-Aspiration Scale (PAS)	1	2	3	4	5	6	7	8
Endoscopic Dysphagia Severity (FEDS)	1	2	3		4	5	6	

Table 5.
Overall estimate of dysphagia severity.

6. Dysphagia complications

Dysphagia and protein-energy malnutrition, being predictors of bad functional recovery, are always associated with a high risk of medical complications. Weaning from mechanical ventilation of such patients is difficult. They have a high risk of purulent-septic complications. At the same time, a risk of sudden death increases [31].

Dysphagia complications are malnutrition, dehydration, weight loss, and respiratory tract obstruction. Aspiration pneumonia is one of the most important complications of dysphagia [32].

When a stroke is complicated with dysphagia, malnutrition occurs 3 times more often than without it. The cases of protein-energy malnutrition in patients suffering a stroke vary from 7% to 15% at acute stage and from 22% to 35% after 2 weeks from the disease onset. Starvation or malnutrition associated with dysphagia activates catabolic processes. Among stroke patients requiring long rehabilitation period, malnutrition can amount to 50%. Malnutrition syndrome is risk factor of pneumonia. It increases sensitivity to oropharyngeal flora, leads to immunity suppression, reduces coughing strength, and affects wakefulness. All these factors complicate rehabilitation procedures [33].

Aspiration is also one of the most dangerous complications of dysphagia. It leads to the respiratory tract obstruction, hypoxia, and aspiration pneumonia [34].

7. Treatment and rehabilitation of dysphagia patients

Neurogenic dysphagia treatment is provided in complex with primary disease treatment. Stroke patients need follow-up and treatment and rehabilitation procedures by multidisciplinary team, including nutritional support, exercises and physiotherapy, logopedic correction, pain control treatment, and psychological correction [9, 15, 35].

Screening test shall always be conducted prior to patient feeding. Patient shall take oral medicines only in the presence or with assistance of medical staff. After taking medicines, a patient shall drink small portions of water. For this purpose, a patient shall be in a semi-sitting position or shall lie on a side with elevated chin; a risk of aspiration is lower in these positions. If even a mild swallowing disorder at pharyngeal phase is observed, it is required to act vice versa: to lower the chin. In this position, the tongue root is pushed backwards, and the epiglottis protective position is improved. This movement compensates for delayed initiation of pharyngeal swallow, as it narrows laryngeal inlet and prevents the bolus passing into the respiratory tract [36].

With nasogastric tube feeding, it is necessary to remember that long-period nasogastric feeding may cause such complications as nasopharyngitis, esophagitis, esophageal stricture, and nasopharynx edema. When dysphagia progression occurs or no swallowing function dynamics have been observed for a long period, a gastrostomy tube is used [37].

Dysphagia patient management, depending on the level of consciousness, reasoned contact, use of a tracheostomy tube, and other factors, shall include the following actions related to examination: [38].

- Medical history taking;
- Swallowing screening test within 3 hours from the moment of admission;
- Examination of the oral cavity, teeth and gums, palpation of the regional lymph nodes;

- Examination of the mouth and pharyngeal mucosa sensitivity;
- Examination of patient's speech apparatus;
- Pharyngeal reflex assessment;
- Testing of the reaction to the tracheostomy tube (when required);
- Testing of the reaction to sanitation of the area above the tracheal cuff (when required);
- Examination of saliva and sputum accumulated in the area above the cuff (when required).

Dysphagia rehabilitation procedures shall include: [39].

- Correct selection of patient feeding pattern;
- Calculation of the caloric value of products with modified consistency and selection of nutritional formulas ensuring nutritional support;
- Selection of food consistency, methods of oral cavity mucosa sensitivity stimulation, swallowing process stimulation and disinhibition, recovery of breath, speech;
- Logopedic exercises therapy aimed at correct positioning, stimulation of active swallowing, normal breathing, recovery and enhancement of functional activity of the muscles involved in the process of swallowing and eating: the muscles of mastication, expression, the tongue muscles;
- Physiotherapeutic treatment methods; in such case, the procedure of choice for neurogenic dysphagia is the larynx electrical stimulation of swallowing reflex;
- Acupuncture;
- Surgical correction (if medically required) aimed at creation of alternative ways for patient feeding;
- Psychological correction;
- Hygienic care of the oral cavity;
- Lifestyle correction aimed at correction or creation of the conditions facilitating independent eating process for patients when the function is diminished or impaired;
- Teaching relatives on feeding skills and complication prevention.

In order to facilitate the impaired process, various methods of swallowing training and retraining are developed. These methods include strengthening exercises, biofeedback stimulation, temperature and taste stimulation [29, 40].

The following rehabilitation methods are used for neurogenic dysphagia patient rehabilitation:

1. Preparatory. Preparation of the oral cavity for swallowing (cleaning and moisturizing with a sponge), removal and installation of removable dentures.

2. "Swallowing enhancement" method. After patient examination, food consistency, which is optimal as for the current moment, is selected. Subsequently, food of various consistency is given, and the volume of food for single administration is increased gradually. At the same time, the required swallow volume, amount of food for single administration, and feeding temperature range are determined. Taste sensation is recovered throughout the rehabilitation period.

3. Replacement therapy method. Nasogastric tube is installed (percutaneous endoscopic gastrostomy is further applied when required). In several cases, parenteral feeding is used.

4. Postural method, which involves the selection of a proper posture required for eating.

5. Training method, which consists of training exercises for strengthening the muscles involved in swallowing process, recovery of swallowing control function.

Complex approach and consistency of dysphagia patients rehabilitation of stroke patients is well-established. Rehabilitation shall be conducted by the members of the multidisciplinary team (MDT) trained on the methods of dysphagia-specific assistance rendering. It is quite important that speech-language pathologists carry out the main works on rehabilitation of neurogenic dysphagia patients. But other members of MDT shall assist speech-language pathologists: physician involved in therapeutic exercises, physiotherapy doctor, as well as patient's relatives.

Physiotherapy tasks: [41, 42].

- Development of adequate afferentation flow by low-frequency electrophonopedic articulation simulation;

- Speech and swallowing management program support;

- Support of non-functioning muscles tonus to prevent their atrophy;

- Prevention of degradation process in the cricoarytenoid joint capsule;

- Recovery and support of CNS regulatory function.

Physiotherapy aimed at electrical stimulation of the larynx and tongue root shall be performed during most of the acute stoke period, when it is medically substantiated.

Approximate current parameters for electrical stimulation:

- Pulse shape: triangular, with a very slow rise;

- Pulse time: 200 ms;

- Pause time: 1,000–7,000 ms (depending on patient's readiness);

- Current intensity: 2.5 mA;
- Time of procedure execution: 30 min;
- Frequency of execution: every day No. 10–15.

The effectiveness of rehabilitation techniques in the treatment of patients after stroke has been shown in a number of studies [4, 10, 18, 29, 37–39]. Various methods of swallowing as part of complex therapy for dysphagia in stroke have shown high efficiency. The best results of swallowing recovery are shown when using integrated approach, include specialized nutritional mixtures with different densities. Recovery was better in patients with pseudobulbar disorders [16, 35]. Involvement of patient's relatives and patient motivation plays a significant role in recovery [4, 9].

8. Dysphagia patients feeding

To perform oral feeding, it is necessary to awaken a patient and seat him/her up before feeding. Make sure a patient stays in a sitting position for 20–30 minutes after the end of oral feeding. First of all, it is necessary to ask patient if he/she wants to take breakfast, lunch and dinner among his/her family members or prefers to eat alone. Anyway, it is necessary to arrange the meal in a comfortable, quiet, and friendly atmosphere, and to put away all unwanted noise sources so that the patient can focus on eating. A patient with difficulty swallowing needs sufficient time for eating. Do not hurry a patient. It is important that a patient feels safe and enjoys the meal while eating.

It is necessary to provide proper positioning of a patient. Correct posture is important to prevent food aspiration while swallowing. When possible, a patient shall sit in an armchair while eating.

When a patient is fed sitting in the armchair, prepare pillows to keep the patient's position, comfortable table and non-slipping carpet before feeding.

Patient shall sit in so that the feet rest on flat surface or on the floor, the body is in vertical positions, and hands are free. If a patient is able to sit on a chair while eating, he/she can also incline forward and lean upon the table. Body inclined forward will prevent the head throwing back. Patient's head shall be on the middle line, not inclined rather than thrown back. The neck shall be slightly (not too much) bent forward to prevent aspiration.

When a patient is not able to keep his/her head position by own efforts, it is necessary to support his/her neck and shoulders from the back to prevent the head throwing back and to help a patient to control his/her tongue position. If, however, the patient's head is inclined too far forward, it is necessary to support his/her chin with the assistant's hand from below or to use special locking collar for the head support.

To prevent aspiration in the process of swallowing, the "chin-to-chest" posture will help; and for patients with unilateral weakness of the tongue muscles, slight turning of the head towards the impaired side while swallowing will be helpful.

When a patient is fed in the bed (if it is impossible to sit him/her in a bedside chair), the patient shall be kept in a comfortable semi-vertical position. For this purpose, raise a patient slightly to the bedhead, supporting him/her with pillows so that the body rests along the middle line. The head and neck shall be inclined forward slightly. The patient's knees shall be bent slightly with a cushion/pillow put underneath.

It is necessary to teach a patient to take food and to lift it to his/her mouth with a hand or both hands. When a patient is not able to suck in liquids, teach him/her to drink from a spoon.

Patient shall be advised to take just a small amount of food or liquid at a time. Teach a patient to lift food or liquid to the middle of his/her mouth, not to a side, and to take food in the mouth using lips, not teeth.

It is quite important to attract patient's attention to the fact that his/her oral cavity shall be absolutely empty after each spoon or piece of food, in order to prevent food accumulation at the side with weak tongue or cheek muscles. Patient shall remove food residuals with a finger after each swallow.

When required, help a patient to clean his/her oral cavity: mucus and saliva accumulated in the mouth shall be removed with wet towel on a regular basis. Remember that the patient's teeth and dentures shall be cleaned minimum twice per day to maintain the oral cavity hygiene.

Do not give a patient drinks together with solid food. In order to reduce the risk of aspiration, drinks shall be given prior to or immediately after eating.

When a patient meets problems with food swallowing, ask him/her to cough up.

Examine the patient's oral cavity after eating. As far as a risk of aspiration still exists for a certain period of time after eating, a patient shall stay in vertical position for 30–40 minutes after the meal.

Do not feed a patient if there are any doubts concerning his/her ability to swallow. In such cases, tube feeding is required.

9. Conclusion

We now know much more about neurogenic dysphagia than we did before. The questions of pathogenesis, clinical picture, diagnostics are well studied. The described approaches in the diagnosis and treatment of neurogenic dysphagia play an important role in clinical practice and are necessary for quality medical care for these patients. Although to date, the level of their evidence remains in the category of cohort studies and expert opinion. This means that we have a lot of interesting work ahead of us and, I hope, important discoveries.

Conflict of interest

No conflict of interest.

Author details

Vadim I. Ershov[1,2]

1 Department of Anesthesiology and Intensive Care, Orenburg State Medical University, Orenburg, Russia

2 University Clinical Research Center of Neurology and Neurosurgery, Orenburg, Russia

*Address all correspondence to: ervad2010@yandex.ru

References

[1] Bakheit AM. Management of neurogenic dysphagia. Postgrad Med J. 2001;77(913):694-699. doi:10.1136/pmj.77.913.694

[2] Belkin A.A, Ershov V.I., Ivanova G.E. Impaired swallowing in case of emergency – postextubation dysphagia. Anestiziologiya i reanimatologiya. 2018;(4):76-82. doi.org/10.17116/anaesthesiology20186304176

[3] Mittal RK. Motor Function of the Pharynx, Esophagus, and its Sphincters. San Rafael (CA): Morgan & Claypool Life Sciences; 2011. Available from: https://www.ncbi.nlm.nih.gov/books/NBK54283/

[4] Reiser MF, Adam A, Avni F, et al. Dysphagia Diagnosis and Treatment. 2012.

[5] Panara K, Ramezanpour Ahangar E, Padalia D. Physiology, Swallowing [Updated 2020 Aug 21]. In: StatPearls [Internet]. Treasure Island (FL): StatPearls Publishing; 2020 Jan-. Available from: https://www.ncbi.nlm.nih.gov/books/NBK541071/

[6] Hall, John E. Guyton and Hall Textbook of Medical Physiology. 11th ed., W B Saunders, 2006

[7] Iordanova R, Reddivari AKR. Neuroanatomy, Medulla Oblongata [Updated 2020 Jul 31]. In: StatPearls [Internet]. Treasure Island (FL): StatPearls Publishing; 2020 Jan-. Available from: https://www.ncbi.nlm.nih.gov/books/NBK551589/

[8] Broniatowski M, Grundfest-Broniatowski S, Tyler DJ, et al. Dynamic laryngotracheal closure for aspiration: a preliminary report. Laryngoscope. 2001;111(11 Pt 1):2032-2040. doi: 10.1097/00005537-200111000-00031.

[9] Powers W.J., Rabinstein A.A., Ackerson T. et al. (2018) 2018 Guidelines for the Early Management of Patients With Acute Ischemic Stroke: A Guideline for Healthcare Professionals From the American Heart Association/American Stroke Association. Stroke, 49(3): 46-110. doi: 10.1161/STR.0000000000000158.

[10] Jones CA, Colletti CM, Ding MC. Post-stroke Dysphagia: Recent Insights and Unanswered Questions. Curr Neurol Neurosci Rep. 2020 Nov 2;20(12):61. doi: 10.1007/s11910-020-01081-z. PMID: 33136216; PMCID: PMC7604228.

[11] Brodsky M.B., Gonzalez-Fernandez M., Shanholtz C., et al. Factors associated with swallowing assessment after oral endotracheal intubation and mechanical ventilation for acute lung injury. PubMed Commons. Medscape. 2014. doi: 10.1513/AnnalsATS.201406-274OC.

[12] Brodsky M.B., Huang M., Shanholtz C., et al. Recovery of Dysphagia Symptoms after Oral Endotracheal Intubation in ARDS Survivors: A 5-Year Longitudinal Study. Ann. Am. Thorac. Soc. 2017; 14(3): 376-383. doi: 10.1513/AnnalsATS.201606-455OC.

[13] Marik PE. Aspiration pneumonitis and aspiration pneumonia. N Engl J Med. 2001 Mar 1; 344(9):665-671. DOI: 10.1056/NEJM200103013440908

[14] Belkin A.A. Syndrome effects of intensive therapy — post intensive care syndrome (PICS). Vestnik Intensivnoy Terapii im. A.I. Saltanova. 2018;2:12-23. DOI: 10.21320/1818-474X-2018-2-12-23

[15] Shaker R, Geenen JE. Management of Dysphagia in Stroke Patients. Gastroenterol Hepatol (N Y). 2011 May;7(5):308-332.

[16] Ershov V.I,. Zdvizhkova S.V., Gonchar-Zaikin A.P., Lozinskaya T.Yu., Kuznetsov G.E., Borodkin I.N., Silkin V.V. The treatment efficiency of disturbed gulping function in patients with ischemic stroke and neurogenous dysfagia in the intensive care unit. S.S. Korsakov Journal of Neurology and Psychiatry 2019;119(7):43 48. DOI: 10.17116/jnevro201911907135

[17] Hammond CAS, Goldstein LB. Cough and Aspiration of Food and Liquids Cough and Aspiration of Food and Liquids Due to Oral-Pharyngeal. Chest. 2006;129:154-168. DOI: 10.1378/chest.129.1_suppl.154S

[18] Bath PM, Woodhouse LJ, Suntrup-Krueger S, Likar R, Koestenberger M, Warusevitane A, Herzog J, Schuttler M, Ragab S, Everton L, Ledl C, Walther E, Saltuari L, Pucks-Faes E, Bocksrucker C, Vosko M, de Broux J, Haase CG, Raginis-Zborowska A, Mistry S, Hamdy S, Dziewas R; for PHADER Investigators. Pharyngeal electrical stimulation for neurogenic dysphagia following stroke, traumatic brain injury or other causes: Main results from the PHADER cohort study. EClinicalMedicine. 2020 Nov 10;28:100608. doi: 10.1016/j.eclinm.2020.100608. PMID: 33294818; PMCID: PMC7700977.

[19] Malandraki G.A., Markaki V., Georgopoulos V.C. et al. Postextubation Dysphagia in Critical Patients: A First Report From the Largest Step-Down Intensive Care Unit in Greece. Am. J. Speech Lang. Pathol. 2016; 25(2): 150-156. DOI: 10.1044/2015_AJSLP-14-0069

[20] Marian T., Dunser M., Citerio G., et al. Are intensive care physicians aware of dysphagia? The MADICU survey results. Intensive Care Med. 2018. DOI: 10.1007/s00134-018-5181-1

[21] Brodsky MB, González-Fernández M, Mendez-Tellez PA, Shanholtz C, Palmer JB, Needham DM. Factors associated with swallowing assessment after oral endotracheal intubation and mechanical ventilation for acute lung injury. Ann Am Thorac Soc. 2014;11(10):1545-1552. doi:10.1513/AnnalsATS.201406-274OC

[22] Thomas S, Sauter W, Starrost U, Pohl M, Mehrholz J. Regaining water swallowing function in the rehabilitation of critically ill patients with intensive-care-unit acquired muscle weakness. Disabil Rehabil. 2017;1-7. doi: 10.1080/09638288.2017.1300341.

[23] Umay E, Eyigor S, Ertekin C, Unlu Z, Selcuk B, Bahat G, Karahan AY, Secil Y, Gurcay E, Kıylioglu N, Keles BY, Giray E, Tikiz C, Gezer IA, Yalıman A, Sen EI, Vural M, Saylam G, Akaltun MS, Sari A, Alicura S, Karaahmet F, Inanir M, Demirhan A, Aydeniz B, Bilgilisoy M, Yuksel A, Ozcete ZA, Calik Y, Alemdaroglu E, Keskin D, Sahin S, Oztekin MF, Sezgin B, Karaahmet O. Best Practice Recommendations for Stroke Patients with Dysphagia: A Delphi-Based Consensus Study of Experts in Turkey-Part II: Rehabilitation. Dysphagia. 2021 Jan 5. doi: 10.1007/s00455-020-10218-8. Epub ahead of print. PMID: 33399995.

[24] Rofes L, Arreola V, C lave P. The Volume- Viscosity Swallow Test for Clinical. Screening of Dysphagia and aspiration. 2012;72:33-42. doi: 10.1159/000339979.

[25] Schepp SK, Tirschwell DL, Miller RM, Longstreth WT. Swallowing screens after acute stroke: a systematic review. Stroke. 2012;43(3):869-871. doi: 10.1161/STROKEAHA.111.638254.

[26] Cullins MJ, Connor NP. Reduced tongue force and functional swallowing changes in a rat model of post stroke dysphagia. Brain Res. 2019 Aug 15;1717:160-166. doi: 10.1016/j.brainres.2019.04.023. Epub 2019 Apr 22. PMID: 31022397; PMCID: PMC6526066.

[27] Macht M, Wimbish T, Clark BJ, et al. Diagnosis and treatment of postextubation dysphagia: Results from a national survey. J Crit Care. 2012;27(6):578-586. DOI: 10.1016/j.jcrc.2012.07.016

[28] Ponfick M., Linden R., Nowak D. Dysphagia - A Common, Transient Symptom in Critical Illness Polyneuropathy: A Fiberoptic Endoscopic Evaluation of Swallowing Study. Crit Care Med. 2014;(C):97416. doi: 10.1097/CCM.0000000000000705.

[29] Kim H.D., Choi J.B., Yoo S.J., Chang M.Y., Lee S.W., Park J.S. Tongue-to-palate resistance training improves tongue strength and oropharyngeal swallowing function in subacute stroke survivors with dysphagia. J Oral Rehabil. 2017;44(1):59-64. DOI: 10.1111/joor.12461

[30] Rodrigues KA, Machado FR, Chiari BM, Rosseti HB, Lorenzon P, Gonalves MIR. Swallowing rehabilitation of dysphagic tracheostomized patients under mechanical ventilation in intensive care units: a feasibility study. Rev Bras Ter Intensiva. 2015;27(1):64-71. doi: 10.5935/0103-507X.20150011

[31] Lang J, Beck J, Zimmermann M, et al. Swallowing disorders as a predictor of unsuccessful extubation: a clinical evaluation. Am J Crit Care. 2008;1 7(6):504-510.

[32] Kim M.J., Park Y.H., Park Y.S., Song Y.H. Associations between prolonged intubation and developing post-extubation dysphagia and aspiration pneumonia in non-neurologic critically ill patients. Ann Rehabil Med. 2015;39(5):763-771. DOI: 10.5535/arm.2015.39.5.763

[33] V.I. Ershov, A.A. Belkin, I.B. Zabolotskikh, V.I. Gorbachev, A.I. Gritsan, K.M. Lebedinskii et al. Russian multicenter observational clinical study "Register of respiratory therapy for patients with stroke (RETAS)": a comparative analysis of the outcomes of stroke during mechanical ventilation. Annals of Critical Care. 2020;4:X–XX. DOI: 10.21320/1818-474X-2020-4-X-XX

[34] Likholetova NV, Gorbachev VI. An analysis of outcomes in respiratory therapy in patients with acute stroke. S.S. Korsakov Journal of Neurology and Psychiatry. 2018;118(6):37-42. (In Russ.). DOI: 10.17116/jnevro20181186137

[35] Ershov V.I., Belkin A.A., Karpets A.V. et al. Effciency of a rehabilitation training method by means of special infant formulas in patients with ischemic stroke and neurogenic dysphagia as part of combined therapy. Nevrologiya, neiropsikhiatriya, psikhosomatika. 2019;11(2):65-70. https://doi.org/10.14412/2074-2711-2019-2-65-70

[36] Lynch Y.T., Clark B.J., Macht M., et al. The accuracy of the bedside swallowing evaluation for detecting aspiration in survivors of acute respiratory failure. J. Crit. Care. 2017; 39: 143-148. DOI: 10.1016/j.jcrc.2017.02.013

[37] Park HS, Oh DH, Yoon T, Park JS. Effect of effortful swallowing training on tongue strength and oropharyngeal swallowing function in stroke patients with dysphagia: a double-blind, randomized controlled trial. Int J Lang Commun Disord. 2019 May;54(3):479-484. doi: 10.1111/1460-6984.12453. Epub 2019 Jan 28. PMID: 30693627.

[38] Park JW, Kim Y, Oh JC, Lee HJ. Effortful swallowing training combined with electrical stimulation in post-stroke dysphagia: a randomized controlled study. Dysphagia. 2012 Dec;27(4):521-527. doi: 10.1007/s00455-012-9403-3. Epub 2012 Mar 24. PMID: 22447240.

[39] Bath PM, Lee HS, Everton LF. Swallowing therapy for dysphagia in acute and subacute stroke. Cochrane Database Syst Rev. 2018 Oct 30;10(10):CD000323. doi: 10.1002/14651858.CD000323.pub3. PMID: 30376602; PMCID: PMC6516809.

[40] Langhorne P, Collier JM, Bate PJ, Thuy MN, Bernhardt J. Very early versus delayed mobilisation after stroke. Cochrane Database Syst Rev. 2018 Oct 16;10(10):CD006187. doi: 10.1002/14651858.CD006187.pub3. PMID: 30321906; PMCID: PMC6517132.

[41] Carnaby GD, LaGorio L, Silliman S, Crary M. Exercise-based swallowing intervention (McNeill Dysphagia Therapy) with adjunctive NMES to treat dysphagia post-stroke: A double-blind placebo-controlled trial. J Oral Rehabil. 2020 Apr;47(4):501-510. doi: 10.1111/joor.12928. Epub 2020 Jan 19. PMID: 31880338; PMCID: PMC7067660.

[42] Andrade JS, Souza WWOJ, Paranhos LR, Domenis DR, César CPHAR. Efeitos da Terapia da Fala em Pacientes Internados com Disfagia Pós-Acidente Cerebrovascular: Revisão Sistemática de Estudos Observacionais [Effects of Speech Therapy in Hospitalized Patients with Post-Stroke Dysphagia: A Systematic Review of Observational Studies]. Acta Med Port. 2017 Dec 29;30(12):870-881. Portuguese. doi: 10.20344/amp.9183. Epub 2017 Dec 29. PMID: 29364800.

Chapter 7

The Interprofessional Clinical and Therapeutic Team Strategy to Manage Spinal Cord Injuries

Adele Jordaan, Mariette Swanepoel, Yvonne Paul and Terry Jeremy Ellapen

Abstract

A popular comorbidity of spinal cord injuries is physical deconditioning that frequently prejudice the person to increased risk for secondary non-communicable diseases, such as non-dependent insulin diabetes mellitus, cardiovascular diseases, respiratory diseases, cardiorespiratory diseases, obesity, osteoporosis, arthritis and osteoarthritis. Clinical literature has shown that spinal cord injured individuals have a poor cardiometabolic risk profile that amplifies the likelihood of secondary non-communicable diseases. Components of physical deconditioning include muscle atrophy, decreased aerobic capacity, inflexibility and diminished muscle and endurance. Another problem associated with spinal cord injuries is reliance or dependence on others. The combination of poor physical conditioning and dependence on others often adversely impacts on the individual's quality of life, limiting their social interaction with others. The adherence to habitual physical activity and exercises has shown to increase conditioning status, improve health and wellbeing, increase independence, and improve confidence and self-image and successful re-integration in community. Therefore it is of paramount importance to increase awareness of the benefits of habitual physical activity and exercise to spinal cord injured patients, medical and clinical practitioners, family and friends. This chapter intends to highlight the health benefits of habitual physical activity in relation to selected secondary non-communicable diseases, and, the importance of interprofessional clinical and therapeutic team strategy to improve the spinal cord injured individuals' quality of life.

Keywords: cardiovascular diseases, exercise, interprofessional healthcare strategy, non-insulin dependent diabetes mellitus, obesity, physical activity, spinal cord injury

1. Introduction

The changes in the spinal cord injured individuals' lifestyle adversely influence their physiological functioning [1, 2]. These individuals generally spend most time sitting that diminishes their physical activity levels, which consequently lowers their energy metabolism. Literature has illustrated that prolonged sitting reduces high density lipid cholesterol (HDL-C) whilst simultaneously adversely increasing the following kinanthropometric (body mass, fat mass, body mass index, waist circumference) and metabolic risk factors (elevated systolic blood pressure, fasting insulin and triglycerides levels) [3–5]. Jordaan and Farrow et al. reported that there is an upsurge in a sub-category of metabolic syndrome among spinal cord injured individuals that being cardiometabolic diseases [2, 6]. Cardiometabolic diseases entail non-insulin dependent diabetes mellitus, renal failure, cardiovascular diseases (especially hypertension) and dyslipidaemia [2]. Considering the paucity of awareness of the clinical therapeutic benefits of habitual physical activity and exercise rehabilitation towards spinal cord injuries, this chapter intends to review empirical literature associate with this topic. A secondary aim is to demonstrate the need for an interprofessional clinical and therapeutic team strategy to enhance the wellbeing and quality of life of the spinal cord injured individuals.

2. The clinical disadvantages that spinal cord injured individuals' experience because of habitual physical inactivity

In this sub-section the authors will describe the altered metabolic profile, body composition, physical capacity, muscle strength and functional capabilities of spinal cord injured individuals. After sustaining the unfortunate occurrence of a spinal cord injury, most individuals become physical inactive (sedentary) which lowers their metabolism, which is pragmatically evident in their metamorphosis of their body composition [7, 8]. Hick *et al* reported that many spinal cord injured individuals become obese (excessive body fat content) and develop obesity-related pathologies, which include non-insulin diabetes mellitus and cardiovascular diseases [9]. Markers of obesity are increased body mass index (beyond 30kg/m^2) and waist-to-hip ratio circumferences (males beyond 0.8 and females 0.7) [10]. Physical inactivity after spinal cord injury with normal energy consumption results in an increased body fat mass and diminished lean muscle mass (muscle atrophy) from disuse [9, 11]. Fisher *et al* reported that spinal cord injured individuals who are habitually physically active and/or exercise, increase their metabolism, which expends more energy, thereby lowering body mass, fat mass and maintains lean muscle mass [11]. Resistance training has proven to be especially helpful to maintain and/or restore loss of muscle mass, as well aid with the reduction of fat mass [2].

Obese individuals muscle cells become insensitive to identify their endogenous insulin; therefore they cannot enter the cells, which prevent the insulin from converting the glucose to glycogen. Sometimes the obese person may become insulin resistant. The obese person is in a state of hyperglycemia. Rajan *et al.* postulated that 66% of spinal cord injured individuals, who are obese, find themselves susceptible to obesity-related pathologies [12]. Obese persons have increased levels of low density lipoprotein cholesterol (LDL-C), which is associated with hypertension (elevated blood pressure) and enlarged atria and ventricles. These cardiovascular morphological adaptations adversely impact the functioning of the heart, leading to various secondary cardiovascular diseases [13]. Clinical literature indicates that spinal cord injured individuals have low HDL-C and elevated LDL-C that increases the risk of atherosclerosis [2, 14, 15]. Tanhoffer *et al* reported that diminished HDL-C levels are a consequence of physical inactivity among spinal cord injured individuals, whilst physical active individuals maintain a high HDL-C and lower LDL-C levels that limit the occurrence of cardiovascular diseases [15]. De Groot *et al* suggested that habitual moderate intensity physical activity and/or exercise among spinal cord injured individuals favorably influence their cardiometabolic profiles curtailing the unfortunate incidence of cardiovascular and metabolic diseases [13].

Post spinal cord injury there is inevitably muscle mass loss due decreased physical inactivity, which consequently reduces muscle strength and endurance [16].

The loss of muscle mass and strength has being associated with decreased functional capacity; leading to greater dependence of others thereby negatively impacting on the spinal cord injured individuals' quality of life [2, 9]. Hicks *et al* and Ellapen *et al* reported that spinal cord injured individuals can prevent drastic muscle strength and mass loss (atrophy) by engaging in regular strength exercises such as arm ergometry and circuit resistance exercises [9, 17]. Hicks *et al* contend that high levels of muscle strength and endurance is positive associated with maintaining the spinal cord injured individuals physical work capacity, functional capabilities and social independence [9]. Physical capacity is the measure of the volume of physical work an individual can perform by quantifying their aerobic capacity and power output [2, 9]. Barfield *et al* emphasized that irrespective of the classification of spinal injury, individuals who are habitually physically active and/or exercise at intensities at a sufficient metabolic equivalents (METS) level are capable of increasing their aerobic fitness [18]. Martin Ginis *et al* reported that spinal cord injured individuals tend to play sport at a prolonged higher METS intensity as compared to their injured counterparts who participate only in exercise regimes [16]. Jordaan concurs with Martin Ginis *et al.* and further recommend that these findings are suggestive that participating in sport might be a more effective mode of physical activity for exploiting optimal cardiorespiratory exercise-induced physiological adaptations [2, 19].

3. The clinical advantages that spinal cord injured individuals gain from habitual physical activity and exercise

The need for regular aerobic, strength and flexibility training among spinal cord injured individuals is paramount in their daily personal pursuit to maintain a healthier quality of life.

i. The need for *regular aerobic training,* is important to increase the amount of energy expended thereby lowering the blood glucose level, which will prevent a state of hyperglycemia and non-insulin dependent diabetes mellitus. Van der Scheer *et al* reported that regular aerobic activity diminish hyperglycemia, adipose tissue, triglycerides, LDL-cholesterol while increasing HDL cholesterol levels, which favorably changes their individual's cardiometabolic profile [20]. Additional benefits include loss of excessive body mass, fat mass, body mass index and increased muscle mass (slow twitch muscle fibers) [21]. Torhaug *et al* and Tweedy *et al* concur that the use of arm cranking ergometry, circuit resistance strength training, manual wheelchair propulsion and swimming increase the spinal cord injured individuals aerobic fitness, upper body muscle strength and endurance [22, 23]. Tanhoffer *et al* has documented that spinal cord injured individuals who frequently use manual wheelchairs possess superior cardiorespiratory/aerobic fitness, which precipitates healthier cardiometabolic profiles [15]. This enriched cardiorespiratory adaptation can be viewed as being beneficial to extend upper extremity aerobic training duration, which will escalate calorie expenditure, thereby decreasing body fat. West *et al* has reported that aerobic training complimentary enhances respiratory functioning of spinal injured individual [24].

ii. Habitual circuit training improves the person's muscle strength and endurance and VO_2peak through the utilization of the short-term energy system, which chiefly stimulates fast oxidative glycolytic fibers [17, 21, 25, 26].

iii. Van Straaten *et al* have documented that habitual physical activity and exercise diminishes spinal cord injury inflammation and neuropathic pain, however the exercise-induced-physiological mechanisms are unclear [27].

iv. The need for regular flexibility training reduces stiff tight asymmetrical muscles, which allows for easier movement [17]. Many spinal injured individuals often have muscle contractures that limit their movement. Regular flexibility exercises decreases muscle contractures by increasing their muscle extensibility, joint range of motion and agonist-antagonist force couple relationship [17, 21].

4. Exercise prescription of physical activity and exercise for spinal cord injured patients

Both the World Health Organization and the American College of Sports Medicine (ACSM) have prescribed habitual physical activity and exercise for spinal cord injured individuals [10, 28]. However their frequency and intensities differ. The WHO suggests spinal cord injured individuals exercise at low to moderate intensity at least three times per week for approximately 30 min a day [28]. The exercise session can be solely strength resistance training or aerobic and/or a combination of both. Whilst Martin Ginis *et al* and the ACSM have prescribed that spinal cord injured adults should engage a minimum of 20 minutes of moderate to vigorous intensity aerobic activity at least twice a week, in addition to two strength training sessions per week [16, 28]. Jordaan disagrees with WHO, Martin Ginis *et al* and the ACSM aerobic exercise prescription because she feels that the aforementioned exercise prescription is insufficient [2, 10, 16, 28]. Jordaan rationale is based on the premise that spinal cord injured individuals are usually physically inactive; therefore, their metabolism is very low expending low amounts energy [2]. Jordaan recommends an aerobic exercise regime of 4 days a week to increase the individual's metabolism and consequently increase their energy expenditure [2]. The rationale for the aerobic exercise regime is based on the clinical fact that many spinal cord injured individuals have poor metabolic risk profiles, which increases their unfortunate campaign towards the onset of non-insulin diabetes mellitus, obesity and cardiovascular diseases [3, 4]. Therefore these individual should follow an analogous exercise rehabilitation prescription plan of cardiac patients, provided they don't have any further contra-indications. The aerobic exercise intensity should range between 11-14 on the rate of perceived effort (RPE) Borg Scale and/or 60-75% of heart reserve. Exercise duration should steadily increase from 10-40 minutes per session as per Ehrman *et al* prescription guidelines [29]. Strength training should be performed at least twice per week consisting of three sets with 8-10 repetitions per exercise for each major muscle group as per Martin Ginis *et al* strengthening exercise guidelines [16]. However the strength training should start at 40% of the incumbent's 1RM and steadily progress to 70% following Ehrman *et al* prescription [29]. Flexibility should further be included at least thrice weekly as recommended by Tweedy *et al* [23].

5. Members of an interprofessional clinical and therapeutic team strategy to manage spinal cord injuries

Spinal cord injured individuals have numerous diseases (neuro-musculoskeletal and non-communicable diseases) that are affecting their wellbeing simultaneously [2].

As such these individuals require an interprofessional team of clinical and medical practitioners to manage their health and wellbeing [30]. The medical and clinical management of a spinal cord injured individuals begins as soon as the injury occurs and persist throughout the person's life; pre-hospital immobilization, surgery and post-surgery rehabilitation and aftercare. Generally the interprofessional clinical and therapeutic team includes a physician (medical doctor), pharmacist, physiotherapist, occupational therapist, kinesiotherapist (United States of America) or biokineticist (South Africa and Namibia), rehabilitation nurse, psychologist and nutritionist [2, 31] (**Figure 1**). The medical doctor is the primary healthcare giver who serves as a referral source to the other practitioners [32]. Grogery stated that each member of the interprofessional team must acknowledge and respect each profession's scope of expertise to ensure success [33]. Due to focus of this book being on the effects of physical therapy on neurological pathology, this sub-section will concentrate on contributions of physical and exercise therapy to management of spinal cord injured individuals.

5.1 Medical doctor/physician

The speciality of the physicians involved in the management of spinal cord injured individuals depends on the time post-injury (that being phase of management and type of injury). During the surgical phase the emergency medical surgeon, anaesthesiologist, neurosurgeon, orthopaedic surgeon is needed. Post-surgery during the rehabilitation phase a pulmonologist, physiatrist, urologist

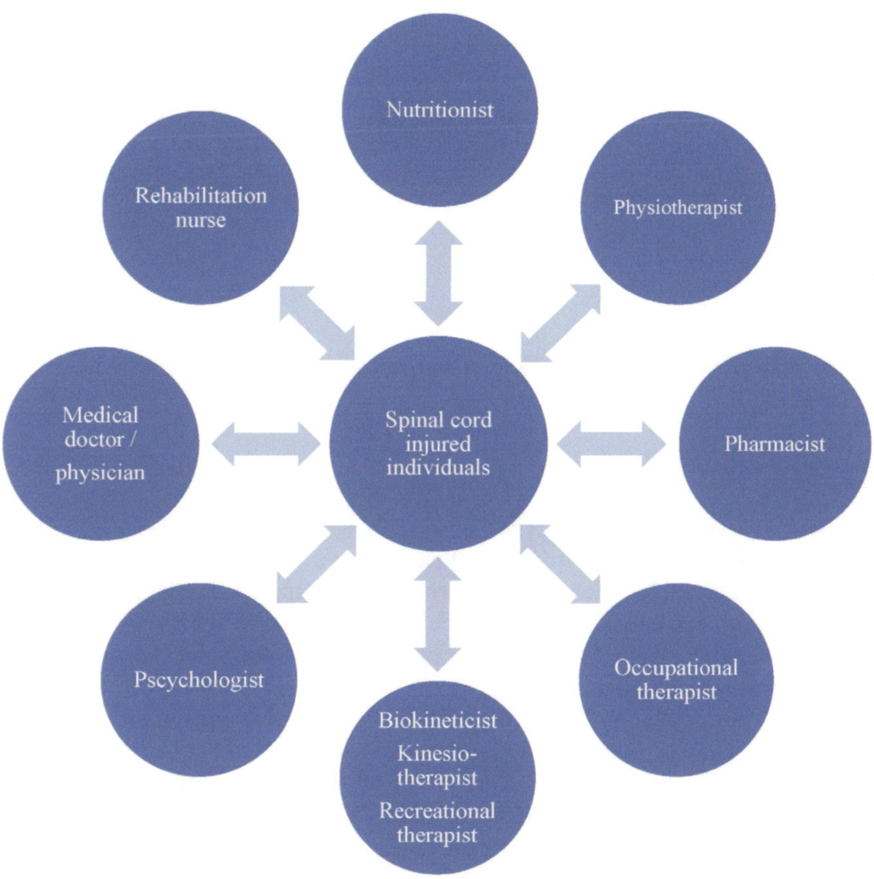

Figure 1.
The interprofessional clinical and therapeutic team supporting a spinal cord injured individual

and a rehabilitation medicine specialist is needed. The aforementioned medical doctors all have significant roles to play in the successful management of spinal cord injured individuals, who needs to comply with their directives [34]. The consulting medical doctor and/or physician general serves as the source of referrals for physiotherapy and exercise therapy (biokinetics and kinesiotherapy).

5.2 Rehabilitation nurse

The rehabilitation nurse has many responsibilities covering a range of clinical and therapeutic functions, such as patient personal hygiene care, person compliance to short; intermediate and long terms healthcare goals which overlaps with many of the therapeutic practitioners scope of professions. Many rehabilitation nurses are present 24 hours, seven days a week, thereby placing them the most admirable position to serve as the coordinators of the interprofessional clinical and therapeutic team because they interact all the clinical and rehabilitative practitioners [35].

5.3 Nutritionist

The significance of good nutritional advice is of paramount value because of the increased risks associated; both malnutrition, (during early post-injury period) and, later obesity that becomes common co-morbidity among spinal cord injured people. Good nutritional choices and habits play a fundamental role to achieve and maintain body mass control, bladder and bowel management, augment immune system function and skin integrity [36]. Collaborative regular monitoring of body mass, body mass index, lean muscle mass and percent body fat mass between the exercise therapist (biokineticist and/or kinesiotherapist) and dietary intake by the nutritionist significantly contribute to assist the spinal cord injured individual maintain optimal body, lean muscle mass and percent body fat.

5.4 Pharmacist

Pharmacist input into the management of spinal cord injured individuals involves medication review of risks that medication can produce to the health of the person and medication prescription [37].

5.5 Physiotherapist

The scope of profession of Physiotherapy spans from intensive in-hospital care, orthopedics, non-communicable diseases, neurology, obstetrics and gynecology rehabilitation [2, 38]. Physiotherapists can manage a variety of concerns of spinal cord injured individual that include diminished respiratory functioning, muscle weakness and contractures, poor somatosensation, reduced mobility, misaligned posture, and deteriorating fitness [35, 39, 40]. The physiotherapists will prescribe physical activity starting from post-surgery confirmed to bed, then bed mobility, transfers maneuvers (from bed to chair, bed to standing and return manoeuvers to bed), assisted gait movement, wheelchair mobility, and upper limb functioning and strengthening. Although a physiotherapist can perform these important tasks other specialists are requested to assist with physical activity and exercise therapy. The physiotherapist may enlist the assistance of a biokineticist (South Africa and Namibia) or kinesiotherapist (United States of America and Canada) to prescribe and monitor stretch, strengthening and aerobic exercises.

In larger spinal cord rehabilitation centers, different movement therapists such biokineticist, kinesiotherapist and recreational therapist may form part of the multi-disciplinary team. Ellapen *et al.* (2018) reported that biokineticists are rehabilitation exercise expertise because their formative tertiary education is Exercise Science and Exercise Physiology [41]. Strydom *et al* and Lawrason *et al* reported that many patients prefer recreational therapeutic physical activities such as sport, games, fishing, gardening, arts and crafts instead of clinical exercise therapy regimes, which on occasion necessitates the referral to recreational therapists [42, 43]. Harvey recommends that physiotherapists should concentrate their efforts to assist spinal cord injured individual to walk with and without assistance, push a manual wheelchair and being able to independently transfer or relocate themselves from one position to another to re-acclimatize themselves to daily living [39].

5.6 Occupational therapist

Pillanstrini *et al* describe the profession of Occupational Therapy as the skilled paramedical treatment, which helps the person to accomplish independence and success in all aspects of their daily lifestyle [44]. The occupational therapist assist spinal cord injured people to re-adjust to their social and physical living environments [44]. De Wit *et al* suggest that the fundamental focus of occupational therapist is the re-acclimatization of activities of daily living through home-based activities, sensory, perceptual and cognitive exercises [45]. Occupational therapists can also assist spinal cord injured individuals who want to return to their careers by re-acclimatizing them to their work-environments, which an aspect that warrants more emphasizes.

5.7 Kinesiotherapist

Kinesiotherapy is an American and Canadian exercise therapy profession that subscribes to the solicitation of scientific, evidence based human movement physical activity and exercise principles aimed to recover the individual's muscular strength and endurance and movement capabilities of patients with functional kinesiological limitations, and individuals who need protracted physical conditioning [46, 47]. A kinesiotherapist functions within the professional association of the American Kinesiotherapy Association. These exercise therapists can assist persons in both the pathogenic and fortogenic healthcare paradigms.

5.8 Biokineticist

A biokineticist is a specialized exercise therapist who functions within the professional association of Health Professions Council of South Africa (HPCSA) and/or the Namibian Health Professions Council (NHPC) [48, 49]. This profession is concerned with final-phase rehabilitation and preventative exercise therapy in the pathogenic healthcare paradigm and the promotion of health and wellbeing in the fortogenic healthcare paradigm [50]. Through individualized physical activity and exercise programme prescription a biokineticist is able to improve the health and wellbeing of a spinal cord injured individual. A biokineticist intends to enhance the physical and physiological status and wellbeing of a patient through an exercise regime in dual context of clinical pathology as well as performance enhancement [42]. Due to the host of non-communicable diseases co-morbidities that affect spinal cord injured individuals the expertise of biokineticists is extremely valuable to curtail their pathogenesis.

5.9 Psychologist

Clinical psychologists focus their efforts to prevent and rehabilitate a variety of psychological problems affecting individuals and families post spinal injury. The psychologist may select various psychological counseling techniques, intended to enhance their spinal cord injured individuals sense of control over these problems, as well as become acquaint with resources that they may employ to overcome their problems. The psychologist also assists the spinal cord injured individuals family to deal with the traumatic event. On occasion the attending psychologist may refer the patient to a neuropsychologist and/or psychiatrist when traditional psychological counseling is inadequate to manage the individuals' psychological problems [35]. Neuropsychologists can play a pivotal role in helping spinal cord injured individuals to address cognition dysfunction that only surface once rehabilitation begins [51].

6. The collaborative interprofessional team strategies to holistic wellbeing of spinal cord injured individuals

The efficacious healthcare management of spinal cord injured individuals necessitates a combination a clinical and therapeutic team approach [35]. Ferguson reported that there three types of interprofessional clinical and therapeutic team strategies can be adopted; multidisciplinary, interdisciplinary and transdisciplinary [52]. Although these terms are interchangeable used to highlight the collaborative nature of inter-professions within the clinical and therapeutic fraternities, there are distinct differences among them [51].

6.1 Multidisciplinary

Jefferies and Chan describe the multidisciplinary team strategy as the elementary mechanism with demarcated professional boundaries involved in holistic healthcare for patients throughout their pathological prognosis, transcending across the primary, secondary and tertiary healthcare phases [53]. The multidisciplinary team comprise of clinical and therapeutic practitioners who coordinate the contribution with little to no overlap. Each profession functions independently, but analogous towards a shared goal; acknowledging each other's contributions towards the mutual success [54]. Each profession drafts individual patient progress reports, which is shared at regular team meetings and as such does not emphasize an integrated approach to care.

6.2 Interdisciplinary

In the interdisciplinary approach, there is an overlap in practice among the practitioners towards a mutual goal within the singular unified management plan. As opposed to the multidisciplinary approach, each practitioner builds on the other's expertise to achieve mutual success. The spinal cord injured individuals progress is communicated through written reports at regular team meetings; however these reports review the overall patient goals and progress rather than individual profession goals and progress [34]. The interdisciplinary team is popular among inpatient spinal cord injury rehabilitation centers. This approach is based on respect of each profession and person and the wellbeing of the patient is of primary concern.

6.3 Transdisciplinary

Among the transdisciplinary team approach is common overlapping of responsibilities across healthcare professions, which insists on optimal communication, co-operation and interaction among practitioners. Clinical and therapeutic practitioners mutually communicate, exchange strategies and reciprocally function. In this approach, there is no hierarchy among practitioners. There is a high level of respect, co-operation and communication among practitioners [35]. The entwined nature of transdisciplinary team approach has the capacity to broaden the skill sets of each practitioner within the team because of their interaction with each. However this team has the potential to be most explosive because the overlap in responsibilities could be mistaken as disrespect for a particular discipline.

Kirshblum and Fergusson reported that the integrated nature of interdisciplinary and transdisciplinary teams is the fundamental difference between these strategic team approaches as opposed to the multidisciplinary team, which does not emphasize an assimilated approach to care [53, 54]. The interdisciplinary clinical and therapeutic team strategy towards spinal cord injured individuals has proven to be most effectiveness among the three team approaches [55].

7. Conclusion

This chapter highlights the need and importance of habitual physical activity and exercise to assist the spinal cord injured individual maintain a healthy life free from non-communicable diseases and secondary cardiorespiratory pathologies. Further the effectiveness of an interprofessional clinical and therapeutic strategy should be careful considered to help manage the lifestyle of the spinal cord injured individual.

Acknowledgements

The authors would like to thank the financial contribution of Tshwane University of Technology towards the publication of this chapter

Conflict of interest

The authors declare no conflict of interest

Author details

Adele Jordaan[1], Mariette Swanepoel[1], Yvonne Paul[2] and Terry Jeremy Ellapen[2*]

1 North-West University, Potchefstroom, South Africa

2 Tshwane University of Technology, Pretoria-West, South Africa

*Address all correspondence to: tellapen1@yahoo.com

References

[1] Bassett RL, Ginis KAM. Risky business: the effects of an individualized health information intervention on health risk perceptions and leisure time physical activity among people with spinal cord injury. *Disability & Health journal*. 2011;**4**(3):165-176

[2] Jordaan A. Physical activity prescription for the prevention of metabolic disease after a spinal cord injury: A systematic review. Unpublished Master's Thesis. North-West University, Potchefstroom, South Africa, 2018.

[3] Manns PJ, Dunstan DW, Owen N, Healy GN. Addressing the non-exercise part of the activity continuum: a more realistic and achievable approach to activity programming for adults with mobility disability. *Physical Therapy*, 2012; 92(4):614-625.

[4] Myers J, Lee M, Kiratli J. Cardiovascular disease in spinal cord injury. *American Journal of Physical Medicine & Rehabilitation*. 2007;**86**(2):1-11

[5] Thorp AA, Healy GN, Owen N, Salmon J, Ball K, Shaw JE, et al. Deleterious associations of sitting time and television viewing time with cardiometabolic risk biomarkers: AusDiab 2004-2005. *Diabetes Care*. 2010;**33**(2):327-334

[6] Farrow M, Nightingale TE, Maher J, McKay CD, Thompson, D, Bilzon, JLJ. (2020). Effects of exercise on cardiometabolic risk factors in adults with chronic spinal cord injury: A systematic review. Achieves of Physical Medicine and Rehabilitation, S0003-9993(20) 30283-5. https://www. doi:10.1016/j.apmr.2020.04.020

[7] Fernhall B, Heffernan K, Jae SY, Hendrick B. Health Implications Of Physical Activity In Individuals With Spinal Cord Injury: A Literature Review. *Journal for Health Human Services*. 2008;**30**:468-502

[8] Baumann WA, Spungen AM. Coronary Heart Disease In Individuals With Spinal Cord Injury: Assessment Of Risk Factors. *Spinal Cord*. 2008;**46**:466-476

[9] Hicks AL, Martin Ginis KA, Pelletier CA, Ditor DS, Foulon B, Wolfe DL. The Effects of Exercise Training On Physical Capacity, Strength, Body Composition and Functional Performance among Adults with Spinal Cord Injury: A Systematic Review. *Spinal Cord*. 2011;**49**:1103-1127

[10] ACSM (American College of Sport Medicine). ACSM's guidelines for exercise testing and prescription. 10th Edition. Lippincott Williams and Wilkins. Philadelphia, 2017.

[11] Fisher JA, Mcnelis MA, Gorgey AS, Dolbow DR, Goetz LL. Does upper extremity training influence body composition after spinal cord injury? *Aging and Disease*. 2015;**6**(4):271-281

[12] Rajan S, Mcneely MJ, Warms C, Goldstein B. Clinical Assessment and Management of Obesity in Individuals with Spinal Cord Injury: A Review. *Journal of Spinal Cord Medicine*. 2008;**31**:361-372

[13] De Groot S, Post MW, Snoek GJ, Schuitemaker M, Der Woude V. Longitudinal association between lifestyle and coronary heart disease risk factors among individuals with spinal cord injury. *Spinal Cord*. 2013;**51**:314-318

[14] Vichiansiri R, Saengsuwan J, Manimmanakorn N, Patpiya S, Preeda A, Samerduen K, et al. The prevalence of dyslipidaemia in patients with spinal cord lesion in Thailand. *Cholesterol*. 2012:1-6

[15] Tanhoffer AIP, Ferreira MB, Abe S, Henneberg R, Hauser AB, Nailwaiko K, Tanhoffer RA, Fernandes LC. Blood profile and general health status in sedentary and physically active individuals with spinal cord injury. *Journal of Exercise Physiology*, 2016; 19(2):76-83.

[16] Martin Ginis KA, Hicks AL, Latimer AE, Warburton DER, Bourne C, Ditor DS, et al. The Development of Evidence-Informed Physical Activity Guidelines for Adults with Spinal Cord Injury. *Spinal Cord*. 2011;**49**:1088-1096

[17] Ellapen TJ, Hammill HV, Swanepoel M, Strydom GL. The health benefits and constraints of exercise therapy for wheelchair users: A clinical commentary. *African Journal of Disability, 2017; 6: 337a*

[18] Barfield J, Malone L, Arbo C, Jung A. Exercise Intensity during wheelchair rugby training. *Journal Sports Sciences*. 2010;**28**:389-398

[19] Martin Ginis KA, Jetha A, Mack DE, Hetz S. Physical Activity and subjective well-being among people with a spinal cord injury. *Spinal Cord*. 2010;**48**:65-72

[20] Van der Scheer JW, De Groot S, Posetma K, Veerger DHE, Van der Woude LHV. Low-intensity wheel chair training in inactive people with long term spinal cord injury. *American Journal of Physical Medicine and Rehabilitation. 2015*;**94**(11):975-986

[21] McArdle WD, Katch FI, Katch VL. *Exercise Physiology: Nutrition, Energy and Human Performance* (7th Ed.) Lippincott Williams & Wilkins, 2012

[22] Torhaug T, Brurok B, Hoff J, Helgerud J, Leivseth G. 'The effect from maximal bench press strength training on work economy during wheelchair propulsion in men with spinal cord injury', *Spinal Cord,* 2016; 54(10), 838-842.

[23] Tweedy SM, Beckman EM, Geraghty TJ, Theisen D, Perret C, Harvey LA, et al. Exercise And Sports Science Australia (ESSA) Position statement on exercise and spinal cord injury. *Journal of Science and Medicine in Sport*. 2016;**1283**:1-8

[24] West CR, Gee CM, Voss C, Hubli M, Currie KD, Schmid J, Krassioukov AV. Cardiovascular control, autonomic function and elite endurance performance in spinal cord injury. *Scandinavian Journal of Medicine and Science in Sports*, 2015; 25, 476-485.

[25] Kressler J, Burns PA, Betancourt L. Circuit training and protein supplementation in persons with chronic tetraplegia. *Medicine and Science in Sports and Exercise*. 2014;**46**(7):1277-1284

[26] Zolot J, Rosenberg K. Wheelchair bound patients who exercise can prevent further disabilities. *American Journal of Nursing*. 2016;**116**(6):69-70

[27] Van Straaten MG, Cloud BA, Morrow MM. Effectiveness of home exercise on pain, function and strength on manual wheelchair users with spinal cord injury: A high dose shoulder program with telerehabilitation. *Archives of Physical Medicine and Rehabilitation*. 2014;**95**(10):1810-1817

[28] World Health Organization (WHO). *World Report on disability*, World Health Organization, Geneva, 2016

[29] Ehrman JK, Gordon PM, Visich PS, Keteyian ST. Clinical Exercise Physiology, 3rd Ed. Champaign, Illnois. Human Kinetics, 2009.

[30] Fehlings MG, Cadotte DW, Fehlings LN. A series of systematic reviews on the treatment of acute spinal cord injury: A foundation for the best medical practice. *Journal of Neurotrauma*. 2011;**28**:1329-1333

[31] Godney J, Reinhardt JD, Haig AJ, Li J. Developing post-disaster physical rehabilitation: role of the world health organization liaison sub-committee on rehabilitation disaster relief of the international society of physical and rehabilitation medicine. *Journal of Rehabilitation Medicine*. 2011;**43**:965-968

[32] Pelletier CA, Ditor DS, Latimer-Cheung AE, Warburton DE, Hicks AL. Exercise Equipment Preferences among Adults with Spinal Cord Injury. *Spinal Cord*. 2014;**52**:874-879

[33] Grogery AS, Dolbow DR, Dolbow JD, Khalil RK, Castillo C, Gater DR. Effects of spinal cord injury on body composition and metabolic profile – Part 1. *The Journal of Spinal Cord Medicine*. 2014;**37**(6):693-702

[34] Dijkers MP & Faotto RM. Team Size in Spinal Cord Injury Inpatient Rehabilitation and Patient Participation in Therapy Sessions: The SCIRehab Project. *The Journal of Spinal Cord Medicine*, 2012; 1;35(6):624-34.

[35] Marshall R & Hasnan N. Chapter.27 Team Based Care. In: Chhabra HS, ISCoS Textbook on Comprehensive Management of Spinal Cord Injuries. *International Spinal Cord Society, 2015*

[36] Momsen A, Rassmussen J, Nielse C, Iversen M, Lund H. Multidisciplinary team care in rehabilitation: an overview of reviews. *Journal of Rehabilitation Medicine*. 2012;**44**(11):901-912

[37] Patel T, Milligan J, Lee J. Medication-related problems in individuals with spinal cord injury in a primary care-based clinic. *The Journal of Spinal Cord Medicine*. 2017;*40*(1):54-61

[38] Aaby A, Ravn SL, Kasch H, Andersen TE. The association of acceptance with quality of life and mental health following spinal cord injury: A systematic review. Spinal Cord. 2020;**58**(2):130-148

[39] Harvey L. Management of Spinal Cord Injuries: A Guide for Physiotherapists. Health Sciences: Elsevier; 2008

[40] De Miguel-Rubio A, Rubio MD, Salazar A, Camacho R, Lucena-Anton D. Effectiveness of virtual reality on functional performance after spinal cord injury: A systematic review and meta-analysis of randomised controlled trials. Journal of Clinical Medicine. 2020;**9**(7) https://doi:10.339./jcm9072065

[41] Ellapen TJ, Paul Y, Swanepoel M, Strydom GL. Do biokineticists transgress on physiotherapists' scope of profession? Evidence-based analysis of two physical rehabilitation disciplines in South Africa. *African Journal for Physical Activity and Health Science*. 2018;**24**(3):316-331

[42] Strydom GL, Wilders CJ, Moss SJ, Bruwer E. A conceptual framework of biokinetic procedures and referral system: an integrated protocol for the various health paradigms. *African Journal for Physical Health Education, Recreation and Dance*. 2009;**15**(4):641-649

[43] Lawrason SVC, Todd KR, Shaw RB, Martin Ginis KA. Physical activity among individuals with spinal cord injury who ambulate: A systematic scoping review. Spinal Cord. 2020;**58**(7):735-745

[44] Pillastrini P, Mugnai R, Bonfiglioli R, Curti S, Mattioli S, Maioli MG, Bazzocchi G, Menarini M, Vannini R, Violante FS. Evaluation of an occupational

[45] De Wit L, Putman K, Lincoln N, Baert I, Berman P, Beyens H, et al. Stroke rehabilitation in Europe. What do physiotherapists and occupational therapists actually do? *Stroke*. 2006;**37**:1483-1489

[46] AKTA (American Kinesiotherapy Association) (2017): Resources, 2017, http://www.akta.org

[47] Paul Y, Swanepoel M, Ellapen TJ, Strydom GL, Wilders C. International comparability of health professions: Bridging the gap between Biokinetics and Kinesiotherapy. *African Journal for Physical Activity and Health Sciences*. 2018;**24**(1):370-383

[48] Health Professions Council of Namibia (HPCN) (2020). https://www.hpcna.com

[49] Health Professions Council of South Africa (HPCSA) (2020). https://www.hpcsa.co.za

[50] Ellapen TJ, Swanepoel M. The Evolution of the Profession of Biokinetics. *South African Journal of Research in Sport Physical Education Recreation*. 2017;**39**(1):41-50

[51] King JC, Nelson TR, Blankenship KJ, Turturro TC, Beck AJ. Rehabilitation team function and prescriptions, referrals, and order writing. Rehabilitation Medicine: Principles and Practice (Edited by Delisa JA). 4th Ed, Lippincott Williams & Wilkins, Philadelphia, 2005

[52] Ferguson M. Multidisciplinary vs. Becoming a More Effective Practitioner: Interdisciplinary Teamwork; 2014 Available from: http://www.socialworkhelper.com/2014/01/14/multidisciplinary-vs-interdisciplinary-teamwork-becoming-effective-practitioner/

[53] Jefferies H, Chan KK. Multidisciplinary team working: is it both holistic and effective? *International Journal of Gynecologic Cancer*. 2004;**14**(2):210-211

[54] Kirshblum S. The Academy of SCI Professionals: Multidisciplinary or Interdisciplinary? *Journal of Spinal Cord Medicine*. 2013;**36**(1):3

[55] Körner M. Interprofessional Teamwork in Medical Rehabilitation: A Comparison of Multidisciplinary and Interdisciplinary Team Approach. *Clinical Rehabilitation*. 2010;**24**(8):745-755

Section 4

Allopathic and Non-Allopathic Medications in Neurological Disorders

Chapter 8

Neurological Phytotherapy by Indigenous People of Rif, Morocco

Noureddine Chaachouay and Lahcen Zidane

Abstract

The Rif region has a rich culture of popular medicine use and valuable medicinal plant practices. This study aimed to assess the potential concerning medicinal plants used in the treatment of neurological diseases. An ethnobotanical survey has been carried out in the Rif for two periods from June 2016 to June 2018. To gather information about indigenous medicinal plants, 520 indigenous people of Rif were interviewed. The data were gathered through semi-structured interviews and free listening, analyzed, and compared. A total of 42 plant species belonging to 37 genera and 23 families were mentioned to be used for treatment by the informants. Lamiaceae was the most commonly reported family in this study area. The most common ailment treated was epilepsy. The preponderance of the herbal remedies was prepared from infusion (53.4%). Leaf was the commonly used plant part (44.3%) and *Marrubium vulgare* L. (29.4%) was the species most commonly prescribed by indigenous healers. The results of this investigation revealed that indigenous communities living in the Rif are still reliant on plants to treat neurological diseases. These reported medicinal species can serve as a source for further investigations on these medicinal plant knowledge and future phytochemical, toxicological, and pharmacological studies.

Keywords: Phytotherapy, medicinal plants, Moroccan Rif, neurological diseases

1. Introduction

The World Health Organization (WHO) estimates that more than one billion people suffer from central and peripheral nervous system disorders globally [1]. The term neurological disorder (ND) applies to any condition that is caused by a dysfunction in part of the brain or nervous system, resulting in physical and/or psychological symptoms [1]. These diseases include Parkinson's disease, schizophrenia, brain tumors, bipolar disorder, epilepsy, neuro infections, Alzheimer's disease, and other dementias, traumatic disorders, and cerebrovascular diseases such as stroke and migraine [2].

Medicinal plants are an important source of active substances that are exploited in the treatment of several sicknesses. In all ancient civilizations and all continents, one finds traces of this use [3]. Thus, even today, despite the progress of pharmacology, the therapeutic use of plants is very present in some countries, especially in developing countries [4, 5].

Today, despite the development of chemical drugs to combat neurological diseases, there is often a return to plants as a source of active ingredients. Besides, an important part of the population, especially in rural areas, prefers medicinal plants, for economic reasons and sometimes because of difficulty in accessing medical care [6].

The rural region of Morocco holds a wide variety of plant species, still offering the possibility to discover very interesting new natural products with potential medicinal value. The Rif region is one of the richest Mediterranean regions in terms of plant diversity, owing to its unique geographical location with geomorphological structures and various climatic. The loss of important medicinal species due to community demand, farming expansion, and deforestation are widely documented by many researchers [7, 8]. This study aimed to investigate local people's use of medicinal plant species used for therapeutic purposes in response to the neurological diseases in the Rif.

2. Materials and methods

2.1 Study area

The research was taken out in the Rif (Northern Morocco) where the Tangier-Tetouan-Al Hoceima region was located. It extends between 34° to 36° of latitude in the North and 4° to 6° of longitude in the East. It is bordered in the North by the Strait of Gibraltar and the Mediterranean Sea, in the South by the Rabat–Sale-Kenitra region and Fez-Meknes region, in the East by the Eastern Region, and in the West by the Atlantic Ocean (**Figure 1**). The total geographical area of the Rif is 11 570 km^2 and the population of the city is about 3 549 512 people with a population density rate of 222.2/km^2 [9].

The study area is characterized by a Mediterranean climate with the highest temperature exceeding 45°C during summer (July–August) and under 0°C during winter (December–January) and the average yearly precipitation ranges from 700 to 1300 mm which falls mainly between October and February [10]. It is mountainous with elevations ranging from 145 to 2.456 (Jbel Tidirhine) meters above mean sea level. This area is dominated by species such as *Tetraclinis articulata* (Vahl)

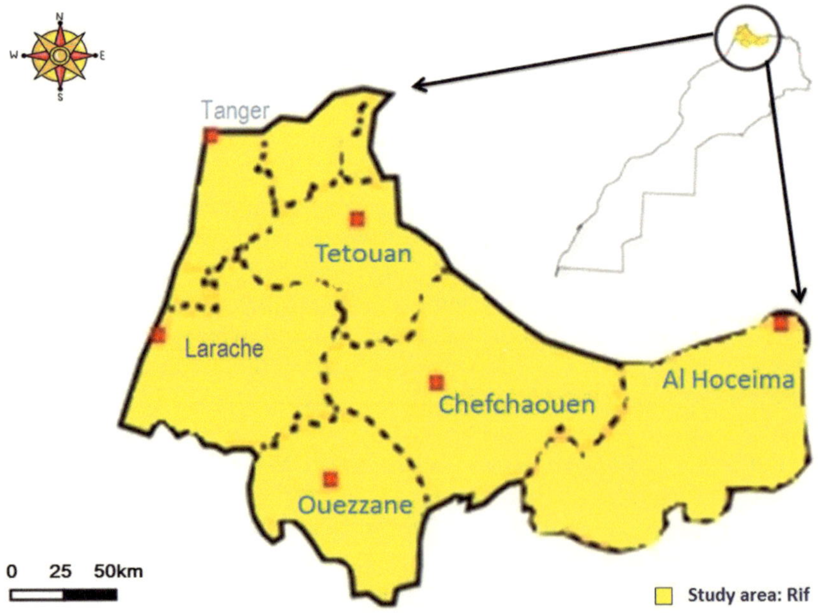

Figure 1.
Map of the study area in Morocco.

Mast., *Cupressus atlantica* Gaussen, *Pinus halepensis* Mill., *Cedrus atlantica* (Endl.) *Quercus suber* L., *Quercus ilex* L., and *Quercus canariensis* Willd. Principally inhabitants of Rif are very much dependent on subsistence agriculture, livestock, and to a minor degree, from forest reserves for their livelihood. Popular medicine is the first choice for the population for health problems, and traditional healers in this area are reputed to have good knowledge of plants and disease treatment [11, 12].

2.2 Methodology

2.2.1 Ethnobotanical survey

Ethnobotanical investigations were carried out from June 30th, 2016 to June 1st, 2018 to collect knowledge on plant species used to treat neurological disorders in the Rif. The techniques employed for data collection were semi-structured interviews [13], free listing, open-ended, group discussion, and noted and recorded with a digital voice recorder. The free survey was designed to collect data on: Socio-demographic information of the informants (gender, age, academic level, and origin of oral health information) and plants used in the treatment of neurological disorders (local names, popular uses, parts used, the form of preparation, method of administration, and posology). Five hundred twenty interviewees aged 17 to 80 were randomly chosen for discussions (cautery installer, farmers, elder people, bonesetters, herbalists, and therapists) in the study area (houses, pharmacies, weekly markets, hospitals, and mosques). By conducting a stratified random sampling, samples were then formed in each of the 28 strata (**Figure 2**), including seven urban communes, and they are put together to make up the overall sample of all informants. The inhabitants in the study area speak Amazigh, Arabic dialects, and therefore, informants were conducted in Arabic dialects or Amazigh. All the documented data was later translated into English.

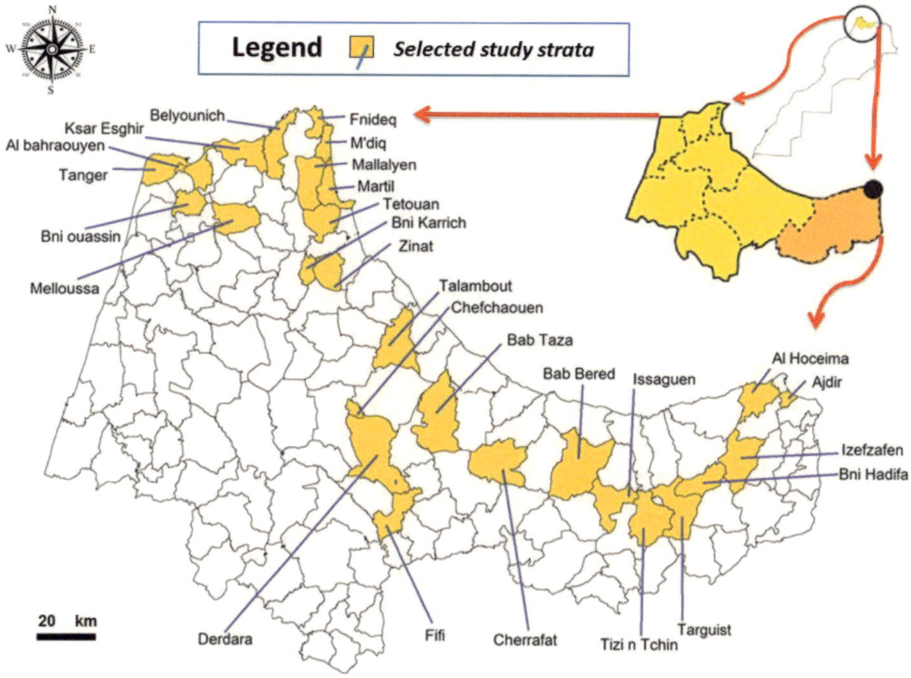

Figure 2.
Distribution of survey points at the study area level.

2.2.2 Plant species collection and identification

Medicinal species being mentioned by the informants were registered with local names and photographed. For each reported plant species, the plant species were accumulated, classified, and voucher specimens were archived. The identification and nomenclature of the collected material vegetal were done first in the field and completed at the *Plant, Animal Productions and Agro-industry Laboratory* by one of the authors using some floristic works of literature as well as: The medicinal plants of Morocco [14], Practical flora of Morocco, tomes I, II and III [14–16] and Catalogs of vascular plants of northern Morocco, including identification keys, tomes I, II [17, 18]. Taxonomy and denominations of species were validated using "The Plant List 2020" database (http://www.theplantlist.org). Voucher specimens have been kept at our University, for future reference.

2.2.3 Data analysis

Data were classified and interpreted by Statistical Package for Social Science (SPSS) version 21 and Microsoft Excel 2010. A representative and quantitative statistical method was adopted to examine the socio-demographic information of the interviewees. All statistical analyses were carried out with Statistical Package for Social Science (SPSS) version 21 and Microsoft Excel 2010.

3. Results

3.1 Demographics of participants

A total of 520 study informants, including 178 herbal sellers, 213 herbalists, 45 pharmacists, 30 midwives, and 54 other traditional healers (bonesetters, fouqaha, cautery installer, farmers, elder people, and nobles), were interrogated using semi-structured surveys and group interviews. In the study area, both sexes are interested in herbal medicine. However, the numbers of females participants were more important (267 informants) than those of male (253 informants). In this study, results showed that the utilization of medicinal species is widespread in all age groups with various percentages. The bulk of informants surveyed were between 40 and 60 years old (232), and over 50 years old (170), while 3 of the informants were the age less than thirty years old. Concerning the educational level, our results revealed that the majority of the informants (77.1%) were uneducated, (19.8%) have primary education, 2.3% have secondary education, and only 0.8% of the informants had high education (**Table 1**).

3.2 Diversity of botanical families

In this study, 42 plant species belonging to 37 genera and 23 families were recorded to be used by indigenous people from the Rif to treat neurological disorders. The scientific names of reported species, their families, vernacular names, plant parts used; method of preparation of each plant species was illustrated in **Table 2**. The family Lamiaceae was designed by the largest number of plant species (6 species), followed by Solanaceae with 4 species, Asteraceae, Brassicaceae, and Fabaceae (3 species each), whereas, the rest of botanical families were represented by one or two species in each.

3.3 Species diversity

The collected information analysis indicates that among the 42 plant species found in the Rif region, 5 medicinal plants are the most used. The specie *Marrubium*

Variables	Categories	Number of informants	Percentages (%)	P-values
Gender	Female	267	51.3	0.857
	Male	253	49.7	
Age groups	< 20 years	6	1.2	0.000
	20–40	112	21.5	
	40–60	232	44.6	
	> 60 years	170	32.7	
Family situation	Married	450	86.5	0.000
	Divorced	32	6.2	
	Widower	23	4.4	
	Single	15	2.9	
Educational level	Illiterate	400	77.1	0.000
	Primary	103	19.8	
	Secondary	12	2.3	
	University	5	0.8	
Income/month	Unemployed	209	42.2	0.000
(Dirham)	250–1500 MAD	192	36.9	
	1500–5000 MAD	80	13.4	
	> 5000 MAD	39	7.5	

Table 1.
Socio-demographic profile of the informants.

vulgare L. was used by 153 informants, followed by *Allium cepa* L. (120), *Matricaria chamomilla* L. (110), *Linum usitatissimum* L. (107), and *Rosmarinus officinalis* L. (103). While the other plants are less used by the local population (**Table 2**).

3.4 Neurological disease categories

Local people of Rif used 42 medicinal plants to treat various neurological disease categories (**Table 3**). The 2 691 use reports were classified into 4 health diseases categories following the International Classification of Primary Care classification system (ICPC) [19]. Most use records were in the category epilepsy (1 142 use reports) and the highest number of plant species used to treat it (21 plant species) followed by headache (950 use reports; 20 plant species) and sciatica (389 use reports; 9 plant species). The last category was associated with meningitis (210 use reports; 6 plant species).

3.5 Plant parts used to treat neurological disorders

In phytotherapy, various plant parts reported particularly leaves, flowers, seeds, roots, fruits, or even whole plant are exploited by the indigenous communities. In this study, the leaf was reported as the dominant plant part used for remedial preparation in their study area (44.3%), followed by bark (11.5%), aerial parts (10.3%), seed (10.2%), bulb (8.8%), fruit (6.6%), root (3.7%), and flower (1%) respectively.

3.6 Methods of preparation

The preparation of herbal remedies needs liquids. The major solvent with the plant was water, but milk, butter, tea and honey, cereal oils were also widely used

Family and Scientific name	Vernacular name	Part used	Preparation mode	Medicinal uses	UR
Amaranthaceae					
Spinacia oleracea L.	Sabanikh	Leaf	Infusion	SC	20
Amaryllidaceae					
Allium cepa L.	Bassla	Bulb	Cataplasm	EL, HC	120
Allium sativum L.	Thoma	Bulb	Cataplasm	EL, HC	70
Asteraceae					
Artemisia herba-alba Asso	Chih	Leaf	Infusion	HC, EL	53
Chrysanthemum coronarium L.	Lgahouan	Leaf	Infusion	HC	28
Matricaria chamomilla L.	Lbabonj	Leaf	Infusion	HC	110
Brassicaceae					
Brassica nigra (L.) K.Koch	Lkhardel	Aerial parts	Cataplasm	SC	23
Brassica oleracea L.	Lmelfof	Aerial parts	Infusion	EL	17
Brassica oleracea var. botrytis L.	Lkrneb	Aerial parts	Infusion	EL, HC	14
Cupressaceae					
Cupressus macrocarpa Hartw.	Sarw	Leaf	Infusion	EL, MG	58
Fabaceae					
Acacia longifolia (Andrews) Willd.	Telh	Root	Decoction	SC	10
Lens culinaris Medik.	Laades	Aerial parts	Infusion	EL, SC, MG	11
Pisum sativum L.	Jelbana	Flower	Infusion	EL, HC	08
Fagaceae					
Quercus canariensis Willd.	Qerrich	Leaf	Cataplasm	HC	60
Quercus suber L.	Bellout	Leaf	Cataplasm	MG	33
Juglandaceae					
Juglans regia L.	Ljawz	Seed	Infusion	El, SC	56
Lamiaceae					
Lavandula dentata L.	Lkhzama	Leaf	Infusion	EL	98
Marrubium vulgare L.	Mrouiate	Leaf	Cataplasm	EL, HC	153
Mentha pulegium L.	Naa Naa	Aerial parts	Infusion	HC	22
Rosmarinus officinalis L.	Azir	Leaf	Infusion	SC	103
Salvia officinalis L.	Salmia	Aerial parts	Infusion	HC, MG	16
Thymus saturejoides Coss.	Zaatar	Aerial parts	Cataplasm	EL, HC	27
Lauraceae					
Cinnamomum zeylanicum Blume	Lquerfa	Bark	Infusion	SC	89

Family and Scientific name	Vernacular name	Part used	Preparation mode	Medicinal uses	UR
Laurus nobilis L.	Rend	Laef	Infusion	HC	75
Linaceae					
Linum usitatissimum L.	Zriat elKtan	Seed	Decoction	EL	107
Myrtaceae					
Myrtus communis L.	Rayhan	Leaf	Decoction	HC	24
Syzygium aromaticum (L.) Merr. & L.M.Perry	Lqronfel	Flower	Decoction	HC, SC	13
Piperaceae					
Piper nigrum L.	Ibzar	Seed	Decoction	HC, SC	12
Poaceae					
Avena sativa L.	Choufan	Seed	Decoction	HC	20
Portulacaceae					
Portulaca oleracea L.	Rejla	Root	Infusion	EL	69
Rosaceae					
Prunus dulcis (Mill.) D.A.Webb	Louz	Fruit	Infusion	EL, MG	16
Rubiaceae					
Coffea arbica L.	Qahwa	Seed	Decoction	EL	26
Rutaceae					
Citrus limon (L.) Osbeck	Limon	Leaf	Infusion	HC	18
Salicaceae					
Salix alba L.	Sefsaf	Leaf	Cataplasm	EL	36
Santalaceae					
Viscum album L.	Dbeq	Bark	Decoction	EL	24
Solanaceae					
Capsicum frutescens L.	Lharra	Fruit	Decoction	HC	30
Datura stramonium L.	Chdeq jmel	Leaf	Decoction	HC	77
Solanum lycopersicum L.	Maticha	Fruit	Infusion	EL	95
Solanum tuberosum L.	Bettata	Aerial parts	Infusion	EL	90
Verbenaceae					
Aloysia citriodora Palau	Louiza	Leaf	Infusion	MG	76
Zingiberaceae					
Curcuma longa L.	Lkharqom	Bark	Decoction	EL	70
Zingiber officinale Roscoe	Skinjbir	Bark	Decoction	SC	63

EL: *Epilepsy,* **HC:** *Headache,* **SC:** *Sciatica,* **MG:** *Meningitis.*

Table 2.
List of medicinal plants used to treat neurological disorders in the Rif, Morocco.

ingredients. No traditional healers reported toxicity associated with their therapies, but in most cases, patients were told to water, milk, butter, tea, and honey, cereal oils were also widely used ingredients. The informants in the present survey were

Categories	Number of taxa	Number of citations
Epilepsy (EL)	21	1 142
Headache (HC)	20	950
Sciatica (SC)	9	389
Meningitis (MG)	6	210

Table 3.
Medicinal plants are used to treat different disease categories.

practicing 3 different types of preparation methods. The results showed that the majority of remedies (53.4%) were prepared from infusion (42.12%), followed by cataplasm (24.4%), and decoction (22.2%).

3.7 Source of medicinal plants

Most of the medicinal plant species recorded in this study grow wild in that region. These species are generally collected at high-mountainous elevation in the highlands surrounding the Rif. Thirteen species (31%) were collected in the wild, 10 plants were cultivated (23.8%), 5 taxa were introduced (11.9%) and 14 (33.3%) were collected as both wild and cultivated.

4. Discussion

Popular medicine practice in the Rif region is diversified and rich. The floristic analysis showed that a total of 42 medicinal species belonging to 37 genera and 23 botanical families were commonly utilized by local people in the therapy of cystitis. The botanical family Lamiaceae was described by the most important number of medicinal plants (6 species). The dominance of Lamiaceae might reflect a rich bioactive ingredient and a wide variety of phytochemical compounds in the species taxa belonging to this family. Scientific studies on these plant families could provide insights into their rich phytoconstituents and understandings of the pharmacological actions of their active compounds. These results are in general agreement with ethnomedicinal inventories which indicated that the most prominent family was Lamiaceae [11, 20–24].

The most commonly used plant species were *Marrubium vulgare* L. the most common significant (29.4%) followed by *Allium cepa* L. (23.1%), *Matricaria chamomilla* L. (21.2%), *Linum usitatissimum* L. (20.5%), and *Rosmarinus officinalis* L. (19.8%). According to many authors, all these plants have phytochemical components with effects on the nervous system [25]. They contain flavonoids, alkaloids, tannins, saponins terpenoids, steroids, and cardiac glycosides. These chemical constituents were considered as the main bioactive compounds of medicinal plants [26]. These chemical contents could be responsible for the traditional use of this plant. Indeed, alkaloids are the most known molecules possessing psychoactive properties [27]. Likewise, some flavonoids, terpenoids, and steroids were quoted to have a psychoactive effect [28, 29]. These chemical constituents intervene to disturb neurotransmitter activities. Moreover, our investigations showed that medicinal plant species that were used by a single or few informants tend to have lower use values than the more prevalent species as shown in **Table 2**. This can imply that some medicinal plant knowledge was maintained and used by a specific traditional healer of Rif's people. However, Tardio et al. [30] stated that a plant with a low use value could be a very important plant for a few people. Therefore, the study of culturally important medicinal plants could provide a deeper understanding of the study area of traditional medicinal practice [31].

The medicinal plants that are widely used by the people of Rif have higher use values than those that are less popular. The highest value of use indicates that plant species are mostly preferred for the study population to treat a given disease. There are 28 plant species highly cited for neurological disorders that should be taken into further consideration through phytochemical, pharmaceutical, and biological studies to evaluate more data regarding their efficacy and authenticity. The present study showed a high degree of agreement among interviewees especially in the categories of epilepsy problems and headache problems.

The reported ailments were grouped into 4 categories based on the information gathered from the interviews. The highest use value was obtained for epilepsy (1 142 use reports, 21 species). These data correspond to those of other ethnopharmacological studies [12, 24, 32–36], which revealed that these pathologies are well-known and treated in the traditional medicine of many countries. The informant consensus values also indicated that the people share the knowledge of the most important medicinal plant species to treat the most frequently encountered neurological diseases in the study area. The agreement information reflects the homogeneity of information provided by different indigenous people regarding medicinal species used to treat a category of ailments. High agreement information is correlated to species that could be efficient in treating a particular ailment [37].

The analyses of results revealed that leaf is the most frequently used part of the plants (44.3%), followed by bark (11.5%), aerial parts (10.3%). The selection of leaves was due to its natural availability, easy gathering, and simplicity in herbal remedy preparation. Besides, the leaves are the seat of the photosynthesis and sometimes the storage of the secondary metabolites responsible for the biological properties of the plant. Similar findings indicated leaf as a major dominant plant part in Morocco [22, 38–41] or Africa [36, 42–44] for herbal medicine preparation.

In the Rif, infusion remains the most dominant method of preparation (41.6%), (53.4%), followed by cataplasm (24.4%), and decoction (22.2%). Infusion is the most common preparation method that is used by traditional healers in other ethnobotanical studies at national and international scales [22–24, 45–48]. These results show that the local population believes in infusion mode and found it suitable for heating the body and disinfecting the plants [49]. On the other hand, the decoction allows collection the most for the active ingredient and attenuates or cancels the toxic effect of certain recipes.

In our study, 68% of the population acquired knowledge about the medicinal use of plants as a remedy for neurological diseases through others' experiences. This reflects the relative transmission of traditional practices from a generation to the next one; the environment and others' experience remain therefore the most effective means to transmit knowledge about medicinal purposes of plants.

The strength of this study is to discover and assess the knowledge and use of medicinal plants in the treatment of neurological diseases in the Rif region of northern Morocco.

5. Conclusion

The present study revealed a very rich indigenous knowledge in terms of traditional herbal medicine used by indigenous people in the study area. The identified natural products used in Rif's communities are a potential source of a novel class of drugs for the treatment of neurological disorders. Based on results, plants scoring high use values should be further tested for their phytochemical and pharmacological investigation. It is important to promote clarity of the general indigenous public, particularly the practitioners of traditional medicine, on the causes, symptoms, and possibilities of treatments for neurological diseases. Therefore, protection measures should be adopted for the conservation of multipurpose and other medicinal plant species. The young generation should be mobilized toward learning ethnomedicinal practices before its extinction.

Acknowledgements

We want to send our sincere gratitude to all the guides and inhabitants of the Rif region for their help. To all sellers of medicinal plants. We also extend our greetings to all those who participated in the success of this work.

Author statement

NC: Carried out field research in the Rif, compiled the literature sources, data analysis, Realization manuscript and evaluation, interpretation and wrote the manuscript, helped in data and made a substantial contribution to data analysis. **LZ:** Performed data analysis and drafted the manuscript; designed the research and identification of plant species. All contributors understand and accepted the final document.

Funding

This study did not take any special grant from funding businesses in the public, commercial, or not-for-profit sectors.

Consent for publication

Consent for publication was obtained from participants.

Declaration of Competing Interests

We guarantee that there is no conflict of interest with any commercial institution concerning the paper.

Ethical Approval and Consent to participate

Consent for this research was given by the Committee for ethical research of the Department of Biology, Ibn Tofail University. Before starting data collection, we received oral informed approval in each case on a site level and then individually before each interview. Informants were also informed that the aims of the investigation were not for financial objectives or other benefits but for academic reasons. Informants provided verbal informed approval to participate in this study; they were free to remove their data at any point in time. Lastly, interviewees have accepted voluntarily the idea and they have agreed to have their names and personal data to be published.

Availability of supporting data

All data collected and analyzed in this paper are included in the article and attached in the form of 'Appendices' as additional files. Plant species are stored in Ibn Tofail University, Kenitra, Morocco.

Appendix A

Questionnaire sheets: Medicinal plants and herbal medicine

Date..

Region ....

Commune..

Survey number..

Informant:

Profession: ....

Sex: Male ☐ Female ☐
Age: { ≤ 20} ☐ {20 - 40} ☐ {40 - 60} ☐ { ≥ 60 ☐
Family situation: Single ☐ Divorced ☐ Widower ☐ Married ☐
Level of study: Illiterate ☐ Primary ☐ Secondary ☐ University ☐
Locality: Nomadic ☐ Town ☐ Village ☐ City ☐
Income / month (MAD): Unemployed ☐ {250 - 1500} ☐ {1500 - 5000} ☐ { ≥ 5000} ☐

Therapeutic practices :

When you feel sick, you address:
To traditional medicine, why?
Effective ☐ Cheapest ☐ Acquisition ☐ Ineffective medication ☐
To modern medicine, why? Effective ☐ More precise ☐ Toxicity of plants ☐
If it is two that it is the first: Traditional medicine ☐ Modern medicine ☐

Vegetal material:

Vernacular name:..
Scientific Name: ....
Plant Type: Spontaneous ☐ Cultivated ☐ Introduced ☐
Use of the plant: Therapeutic ☐ Cosmetic ☐ Other ☐
Harvesting technique: Manual ☐ Mechanical ☐
Harvest Time: Summer ☐ Fall ☐ Winter ☐ Spring ☐ Any year ☐
Drug preparation: Plant alone ☐ Possible association (of plants) ☐
If the association of plants, quote the recipe:..
Use of the plant: Fresh ☐ Desiccated ☐ After treatment ☐
If desiccated, drying method: Sun exposure ☐ In the Shade ☐
Used part: Stem ☐ Flower ☐ Fruit ☐ Seed ☐ Bark ☐ Bulb ☐
Root Rhizome ☐ Leaf ☐ Whole plant ☐ Other combination ☐ ☐

Form of employment: Tisane ☐ Powder ☐ Essential oil ☐ Oily oil ☐ Tincture ☐

Method of preparation: Infusion ☐ Decoction ☐ Cataplasm ☐ Raw ☐ cooked ☐ Other ☐
The dose used: Pinch ☐ Handle ☐ Spoonful ☐
Precise Dose: Quantity in g / glass: .... Quantity in g / liter: .... Other: ....
Administration mode: Oral ☐ Massage ☐ Rinse ☐ Swabbing ☐ Other ☐
Dosage: number of doses per day:
For children: 1time / day ☐ 2time / day ☐ 3time / day ☐ Other ☐
For adults: 1time / day ☐ 2time / day ☐ 3time / day ☐ Other ☐

For older people: 1time / day ☐ 2time / day ☐ 3time / day ☐ Other ☐

Length of Use: One Day ☐ A Week ☐ One month ☐ Until healing ☐

Conservation method: Sheltered from the light ☐ Exposed to light ☐ Other ☐
Expiration date:..

Use :

Diagnosis By: Himself ☐ Doctor ☐ Herbalist ☐ Other ☐
Results: Healing ☐ Improvement ☐ Ineffective ☐
Side effect: .... Toxicity: .... Caution of use: ....

Author details

Noureddine Chaachouay[1*] and Lahcen Zidane[2]

1 Higher education and training school, University Hassan, Settat, Morocco

2 Plant, Animal Productions and Agro-Industry Laboratory, Department of Biology, Faculty of Sciences, Ibn Tofail University, Kenitra, Morocco

*Address all correspondence to: nour.chay@gmail.com

References

[1] WHO. What Are Neurological Disorders, World Health Organization. DOI: http://www.who.int/features/qa/55/en/.2016.

[2] Stephenson J, Nutma E, van der Valk P, Amor S. Inflammation in CNS Neurodegenerative Diseases. Immunology. 2018, 154 (2), 204-219. https://doi.org/10.1111/imm.12922.

[3] Gurib-Fakim A. Medicinal Plants: Traditions of Yesterday and Drugs of Tomorrow. Mol. Aspects Med. 2006, 27 (1), 1-93.

[4] Da Silva V. A, do Nascimento V. T, Soldati G. T, Medeiros M. F. T, Albuquerque U. P. Methods and Techniques, Ethnobiology and Ethnoecology. humana press. De Carvalho, L. M. M. 2011. Ethnobiology, Wiley-Blackwell. 2014.

[5] Chaachouay N, Benkhnigue O, Fadli M, El Ibaoui H, Zidane L. Ethnobotanical and Ethno-pharmacological Studies of Medicinal and Aromatic Plants Used in the Treatment of Metabolic Diseases in the Moroccan Rif. Heliyon. 2019, p e02191.

[6] Organization W. H. World Health Statistics 2010; World Health Organization, 2010.

[7] Benbrahim K. F, Ismaili M, Benbrahim S. F, Tribak A. Problèmes de Dégradation de l'environnement Par La Désertification et La Déforestation: Impact Du Phénomène Au Maroc. Sci. Chang. Planétaires Sécheresse. 2004, 15 (4), 307-320.

[8] Roose É, Sabir M, Arabi M, Morsli B, Mazour M. Soixante Années de Recherches En Coopération Sur l'érosion Hydrique et La Lutte Antiérosive Au Maghreb. Physio-Géo Géographie Phys. Environ. 2012, No. Volume 6, 43-69.

[9] HCP. Haut-Commissariat au Plan, Monographie De La Region Tanger-Tetouan-Al Hoceima', Haut-commissariat au plan, Rabat — Maroc., 2018. DOI: https://www.hcp.ma/region-tanger/Monographie-de-la-region-de-Tanger-Tetouan-Al-Hoceima-2018_a416.html.

[10] DMNM. Direction de la Météorologie Nationale, Maroc. 2018.

[11] Benabid A, Bellakhdar J. Relevés Floristiques et Catalogue Des Plantes Médicinales Dans Le Rif Occidental. Al Biruniya. 1987, 3 (2), 87-120.

[12] Chaachouay N, Benkhnigue O, Zidane L. Ethnobotanical Study Aimed at Investigating the Use of Medicinal Plants to Treat Nervous System Diseases in the Rif of Morocco. J. Chiropr. Med. 2020, 19 (1), 70-81.

[13] Jain, S. K. The Role of Botanist in Folklore Research. Folklore. 1964, 5 (4), 145-150.

[14] Sijelmassi A. Les Plantes Médicinales Du Maroc, 3ème Édition Fennec. Casablanca Moroc 1993.

[15] Fennane M, Tattou M. I, Mathez J, Quézel P. Flore Pratique Du Maroc: Manuel de Détermination Des Plantes Vasculaires. Pteridophyta, Gymnospermae, Angiospermae (Lauraceae-Neuradaceae); Institut scientifique, 1999.

[16] Fennane M, Tattou M. I, Valdés B. Catalogue Des Plantes Vasculaires Rares, Menacées Ou Endémiques Du Maroc; Herbarium Mediterraneum Panormitanum, 1998.

[17] Fennane M, Ibn Tattou M, El Oualidi J. Flore Pratique Du Maroc, Dicotylédones (Pp), Monocotylédones. Trav. L'Institut Sci. Rabat Sér. Bot. 2014, 40.

[18] Valdés B. Catalogue Des Plantes Vasculaires Du Nord Du Maroc, Incluant Des Clés d'identification; Editorial CSIC-CSIC Press. 2002; Vol. 1.

[19] Lamberts H, Wood M. ICPC, International Classification of Primary Care; Oxford University Press, USA, 1987.

[20] Chaachouay N, Zidane L. Ethnomedicinal Studies on Medicinal Plants Used by People of Rif, Morocco. 2019.

[21] Chaachouay N, Benkhnigue O, Fadli M, El Ayadi R, Zidane L. Ethnobotanical Study of Medicinal Plants Used to Treat Osteoarticular Diseases in the Moroccan Rif, Morocco. J. Pharm. Pharmacogn. Res. 2019, 7 (6), 454-470.

[22] Benkhnigue O, Zidane L, Fadli M, Elyacoubi H, Rochdi A, Douira A. Etude Ethnobotanique Des Plantes Médicinales Dans La Région de Mechraâ Bel Ksiri (Région Du Gharb Du Maroc). Acta Bot. Barcinonensia. 2010, 53, 191-216.

[23] Islam M, Ahmad H, Rashid A, Razzaq A, Akhtar N, Khan,I. Weeds and Medicinal Plants of Shawar Valley, District Swat. Pak J Weed Sci Res. 2006, 12 (1-2), 83-88.

[24] Majeed M, Bhatti K. H, Amjad M. S, Abbasi A. M, Bussmann R. W, Nawaz,F, Rashid A, Mehmood A, Mahmood M, Khan W. M. Ethno-Veterinary Uses of Poaceae in Punjab, Pakistan. PloS One 2020, 15 (11), e0241705.

[25] Sucher N. J, Carles M. C. A Pharmacological Basis of Herbal Medicines for Epilepsy. Epilepsy Behav. 2015, 52, 308-318.

[26] Sereme A, Milogo-Rasolodimby J, Guinko S,Nacro M. Propriétés Thérapeutiques Des Plantes à Tanins Du Burkina Faso. Pharmacopée Médecine Tradit. Afr. 2011, 15.

[27] Ujváry I. Psychoactive Natural Products: Overview of Recent Developments. Ann. Ist. Super. Sanita. 2014, 50, 12-27.

[28] Amar M. B. La Polyconsommation de Psychotropes et Les Principales Interactions Pharmacologiques Associées; Centre québécois de lutte aux dépendances. 2007.

[29] Zhang Z.-J. Therapeutic Effects of Herbal Extracts and Constituents in Animal Models of Psychiatric Disorders. Life Sci. 2004, 75 (14), 1659-1699.

[30] Tardío J, Pardo-de-Santayana M. Cultural Importance Indices: A Comparative Analysis Based on the Useful Wild Plants of Southern Cantabria (Northern Spain). Econ. Bot. 2008, 62 (1), 24-39.

[31] Tangjitman K, Wongsawad C, Winijchaiyanan P, Sukkho T, Kamwong K, Pongamornkul W, Trisonthi C. Traditional Knowledge on Medicinal Plant of the Karen in Northern Thailand: A Comparative Study. J. Ethnopharmacol. 2013, 150 (1), 232-243.

[32] Maria M. R, Maria Cristina D, Bucar I, Luís C. Medicinal Plants Used to Treat Neurological Disorders in West Africa: A Case Study with Guinea-Bissau Flora. Am. J. Plant Sci. 2012, 2012.

[33] Saki K, Bahmani M, Rafieian-Kopaei M, Hassanzadazar H, Dehghan K, Bahmani F, Asadzadeh J. The Most Common Native Medicinal Plants Used for Psychiatric and Neurological Disorders in Urmia City, Northwest of Iran. Asian Pac. J. Trop. Dis. 2014, 4, S895–S901.

[34] Parvez M. K. Natural or Plant Products for the Treatment of Neurological Disorders: Current Knowledge. Curr. Drug Metab. 2018, 19 (5), 424-428.

[35] Kinda P. T, Zerbo P, Guenné S, Compaoré M, Ciobica A, Kiendrebeogo M. Medicinal Plants Used

for Neuropsychiatric Disorders Treatment in the Hauts Bassins Region of Burkina Faso. Medicines. 2017, 4 (2), 32.

[36] Mukungu N, Abuga K, Okalebo F, Ingwela R, Mwangi J. Medicinal Plants Used for Management of Malaria among the Luhya Community of Kakamega East Sub-County, Kenya. J. Ethnopharmacol. 2016, 194, 98-107.

[37] Uddin M. Z, Hassan M. A. Determination of Informant Consensus Factor of Ethnomedicinal Plants Used in Kalenga Forest, Bangladesh. Bangladesh J. Plant Taxon. 2014, 21 (1), 83-91.

[38] Chaachouay N, Benkhnigue O, Douira A, Zidane,L. Poisonous Medicinal Plants Used in the Popular Pharmacopoeia of the Rif, Northern Morocco. Toxicon. 2021, pp 24-32.

[39] Chaachouay N, Benkhnigue O, Khamar H, Zidane L. Ethnobotanical Study of Medicinal and Aromatic Plants Used in the Treatment of Genito-Urinary Diseases in the Moroccan Rif. Journal of Materials and Environmental Sciences. 2020, pp 15-29.

[40] Chaachouay N, Douira A, Zidane L. COVID-19, Prevention and Treatment with Herbal Medicine in the Herbal Markets of Salé Prefecture, North-Western Morocco. Eur. J. Integr. Med. 2021, 101285.

[41] Bammi J, Douira A. Les Plantes Médicinales Dans La Forêt de l'achach (Plateau Central, Maroc). 2002.

[42] Asnake S, Teklehaymanot T, Hymete A, Erko B, Giday M. Survey of Medicinal Plants Used to Treat Malaria by Sidama People of Boricha District, Sidama Zone, South Region of Ethiopia. Evid. Based Complement. Alternat. Med. 2016, 2016.

[43] Asase A, Akwetey G. A, Achel D. G. Ethnopharmacological Use of Herbal Remedies for the Treatment of Malaria in the Dangme West District of Ghana. J. Ethnopharmacol. 2010, 129 (3), 367-376.

[44] Nouri J. Étude Floristique et Ethnobotanique Des Plantes Médicinales Au Nord-Ouest de La Tunisie: Cas de La Communauté d'Ouled Sedra. J. Adv. Res. Sci. Technol. 2016, 3 (1), 281-291.

[45] Chaachouay N, Benkhnigue O, El Ibaoui H, El Ayadi R, Zidane L. Medicinal plants used for diabetic problems in the Rif, Morocco. Ethnobotany Research and Applications. 2019.

[46] Chaachouay N, Benkhnigue O, Fadli M, El Ibaoui H, El Ayadi R, Zidane L. Ethnobotanical and Ethnopharmacological Study of Medicinal and Aromatic Plants Used in the Treatment of Respiratory System Disorders in the Moroccan Rif. Ethnobotany Research and Applications. 2019, pp 1-16.

[47] Iqbal M. Vicia Faba Bioassay for Environmental Toxicity Monitoring: A Review. Chemosphere. 2016, 144, 785-802.

[48] Abdurhman N. Ethnobotanical Study of Medicinal Plants Used by Local People in Ofla Wereda, Southern Zone of Tigray Region Ethiopia. Addis Ababa Univ. MSc Thesis 2010.

[49] Lahsissene H, Kahouadji A, Hseini S. Catalogue Des Plantes Medicinales Utilisees Dans La Region de Zaër (Maroc Occidental). Lejeunia Rev. Bot. 2009.

Chapter 9

Pharmacological Modulation of Toll-Like Receptors in Brain Disorders

Tahani K. Alshammari, Nouf M. Alrasheed, Lina Alhushan, Reema Alhoutah, Anfal F. Bin Dayel, Asma S. Alonazi and Musaad A. Alshammari

Abstract

The knowledge regarding pathological and treatment resistance mechanisms involved in the pathology of complex brain disorders is far from understood. The neuroinflammation hypothesis of psychiatric, neurological, and neurodegenerative diseases is well-acknowledged. However, this hypothesis is far from understood. Toll-like receptors (TLRs) family is an innate immunity molecule implicated in neuroinflammation in complex brain disorders. This chapter reviews considerable evidence indicating that activation of endotoxins such as lipopolysaccharide is a common factor. Additionally, we report clinical and preclinical studies highlighting the link between lipopolysaccharide, TLRs, and different types of brain disorders. Also, we review the current pharmacological modulations of TLRs. Hoping we would help in filling our knowledge gaps and highlight potential links to tackle new angles in managing complex brain disorders. This chapter's primary goal is to encourage scientists and researchers to conduct future studies characterizing the nature of endotoxin activation of TLRs in complex brain disorders, filling our knowledge gaps, and finding new treatment strategies.

Keywords: Brain disorders, Toll-like receptors, TLR4, Endotoxins, lipopolysaccharide

1. Introduction

The complex nature of neurodegenerative and psychiatric diseases stems from pathological interactions, among which inflammation [1]. Neuroinflammation is a crucial mechanism involved in the pathogenesis of psychiatric [2] and neurodegenerative diseases [3]. Accumulating evidence indicating that targeting neuroinflammation is an appealing strategy since that inflammatory-related diseases comorbid with brain disorders [4–7]. In preclinical settings, triggering inflammation by administering of endotoxins and other activators are well-acknowledged animal models [8]. Preclinical studies found that attenuating inflammation reduces phenotypic features associated with psychiatric and neurodegenerative disorders. In line with this, clinical studies suggest that treatment with anti-inflammatory medications affects memory, cognition, and mood [9–11].

IntechOpen

Developmental studies have shown that TLRs are essential elements in regulating brain development. Previously, it was reported that both TLR7 and TLR9 are expressed in corticolimbic regions of the developing brain. *In situ* hybridization and PCR studies indicated that TLR7 and TLR9 expression increased significantly in pre and early postnatal stages, whereas the expression reduced as the rodents reached adult developmental stages [12]. Epidemiological reports indicated that exposure to infection at prenatal stages, where the brain and the central nervous system are developing and vulnerable to an unfavorable environment, increases mental illness risk later in life [13, 14]. Inflammatory cytokines involve ubiquitously in modulating different pathways. For instance, it may alter the developing brain epigenetic system, which could be due to excessive glucocorticoids [14]. According to the Danish National Psychiatric Register, prenatal exposure to bacterial infection was linked to schizophrenia. In a set of about 8000 individuals, 1.1% of cases were diagnosed with schizophrenia by their thirties [15]. In line with this, a previous study linked developmental delay and mental retardation to maternal urinary tract infections [16]. On another cohort, the risk of schizophrenia increases in offspring born to mothers diagnosed with reproductive infections during pregnancy [17]. Also, other reports link cytokine-related mechanisms to the pathology of Attention deficit hyperactivity disorder [18, 19]. *In vitro* studies have shown that TLR3, TLR7 and, TLR8 regulate dendritic arborization in an MYD88 dependent signaling. The studies indicated that among these receptors, the TLR8 is the major contributor in regulating dendritic pruning. It further showed that both TLR3 and TLR7 are essential in regulating axonal development. This evidence indicated that the TLR family is vital in modulating proper neuronal development [20].

All these evidences indicate a functional direct link between inflammation and mental illness. This chapter was undertaken to further highlight the association of TLRs, endotoxins, and brain disorders. We also emphasize the diverse role of multiple TLR family members in both nonregenerative and psychiatric diseases. Lastly, we review the pharmacological modulation of TLRs in the context of brain disorders. Aiming this chapter would stimulate future research in characterizing the nature of endotoxin activation of TLRs in complex brain disorders, filling our knowledge gaps, and finding new treatment strategies.

2. The role of endotoxins in mediating brain disorders

In comparison to most bacterial activators of inflammatory cytokines, endotoxins are considered one of the most potent. Mostly, endotoxins are referred to as lipopolysaccharide (LPS) [21]. LPS is a composition of the bacterial cell wall; an elevated level of LPS reaches different biological systems during infections. Administration of LPS to healthy participants induces both the initiation and the transition phases of acute inflammation. Besides, this activation level reaches the transcriptomic level along with the functional and physiological levels [22]. The systemic application of LPS is utilized extensively in pharmacological animal models of brain disorders [23], including Alzheimer's [24], Parkinson's [25], depression [26], and anxiety [27]. This is mainly regarded as the potency in triggering inflammation.

Previous reports indicated that LPS stimulates the aggregations of both amyloid β and tau, a neuropathological feature of Alzheimer's [28]. Treating Tg2576 mice with LPS increases the mRNA level of cytokines in the cortex [29]. In a transgenic animal model of Alzheimer's, the 3xTg-AD mice, administration of LPS trigger pathological changes in microglia populations associated with later on aggregations of hyperphosphorylated tau. Even though the researchers exposed these mice to

LPS at early developmental stages, before the detection of pathological features related to Alzheimer's disease. Additionally, they reported that the aggregation of phosphorylated tau was mediated mechanistically through the activation of the cyclin-dependent kinase 5 (cdk5) [30]. Cdk5 is a member of the cyclin-dependent kinases family. Specifically, they are proline-directed serine–threonine kinases group. Functionally, Cdk5 modulates the cell cycle [31, 32], synaptic wiring, neuronal transmission [33], and neuronal development and survival [34]. In accordance with this, a previous report demonstrated that following the stereotaxic introduction of Aβ in mice, the pharmacological inhibition of Cdk5 using roscovitine resulted in reducing inflammatory and oxidative stress mediators at the mRNA level. Indicating that, Cdk5 is a crucial modulator of neuroinflammation associated with molecular phenotypic features of Alzheimer's disease [35]. Lipopolysaccharide alters the blood–brain barrier transport of amyloid beta protein: a mechanism for inflammation in the progression of Alzheimer's disease [36]. Also, in a transgenic model lacking the NADPH oxidase regulatory gene, the administration of LPS led to molecular and cellular neurodegenerative changes associated with Parkinson's disease [37]. In line with this, the pre-administration with LPS resulted in accelerated aging and Parkinson -related symptoms in a Parkinson's animal model [38]. Describes the main mechanisms involved in the LPS animal models **Table 1**.

In a clinical setting, a previous report indicated that depression and marital distress were significantly associated with an increased LPS, LPS binding protein, and soluble CD14, an LPS co-receptor. Indicating that activation and the translocation of bacterial endotoxin are crucial in mediating mood disorders and stress-related diseases [39]. Functional imaging indicated that individuals exposed to endotoxemia had shown elevated levels of alertness [40], and emotional sensitivity toward visual stimuli [41]. Biochemical changes were observed peripherally, such as elevated stress hormones and inflammation [40, 41], and alterations in the sympathetic nerve's activity [42]. In another clinical study, the cognitive capacity of

Disease model	Phenotypic molecular and behavioral features	Reference
Model of Alzheimer's disease *(Tg2576 mice)*.	• Treating Tg2576 mice with LPS increases the mRNA level of cytokines in the cortex	[29]
Model of Alzheimer's disease *(3xTg-AD mice)*	• Pathological changes in microglia populations. • Aggregations of hyperphosphorylated tau. • Activation of the cyclin-dependent kinase 5 (cdk5).	[30]
LPS administration to a Parkinson's disease animal model. (NOX2-/-)mice	• A loss in dopaminergic neurons. • Oxidative stress and Parkinson-related features.	[37]
Endotoxin-Induced Neuroinflammation Model of Parkinson's Disease.	• Resulted in accelerated aging and Parkinson -related symptoms. • Modify reactive microglia. • Alter the peripheral level of inflammatory cytokines (IL-6, IL-2,TNF-alpha,IFN-gamma)	[38]
Model of Alzheimer's disease.	• The administration of LPS in mice promoted the influx of amyloid beta protein to the brain and reduced their efflux, a unifying feature of Alzheimer's disease.	[36]

Tg2576: Transgenic Tg2576 mice; LPS: lipopolysaccharide; NOX2: NADPH oxidase 2; IL-2: Interleukin 2; IL-6: Interleukin 6; IFN-gamma: Interferon gamma.

Table 1.
Main mechanisms involved in the lipopolysaccharide animal models.

healthy participants exposed to endotoxin systemically was examined. The results suggested that the endotoxin-exposed group exhibited a reduction in cognitive function and reduced capability in processing emotional information compared to the placebo group [43]. Suggesting that short-term exposure to systemic endotoxin has a profound impact on higher cognitive tasks. Disrupted sociability [44], and impaired cognitive capacity are hallmarks of psychiatric disorders [45], mainly schizophrenia, and autism [46, 47]. In another report, a battery of socio-behavioral factors was examined and reported to be functionally linked to the systemic administration of LPS. Indicating a mechanistic link between LPS-inflammation and major depressive disorder [48]. In line with this, the administration of a citalopram, a selective serotonin reuptake inhibitor antidepressant agent, leads to a reduction in fatigue and multiple inflammatory cytokines associated with endotoxins activation [49]. In another clinical setting, the level of circulating endotoxins correlates with the severity of neurodegenerative disorders, including Alzheimer's, sporadic amyotrophic lateral sclerosis (sALS) [50].

3. TLR and brain disorders

Toll-like receptor (TLR) is a family composed of multiple pattern recognition members, and these receptors play a crucial role in mediating and modulating innate immunity [51]. This family has an essential role in modulating and maintaining the microglia and microglia translocation protein activity. Histological studies indicated that multiple members of this family are expressed in the brain [52, 53], gut and blood mononuclear cells [54]. Additionally, these receptors are functionally involved in modulating excitatory [55], and inhibitory neuronal populations [56–58]. These modulations include orchestrating different signaling pathways [20]. Also, a couple of TLRs (TLR2 and TLR9) regulate the enteric nervous system. A previous report has shown that both receptors were detected using histological studies in multiple markers of the enteric nervous system. Upon activation of innate immunity by administration LPS, both members were upregulated in the enteric nervous system. Indicating selective disease activation mechanism [55]. Correspondingly, LPS activation of TLR4 leads to stimulation of cytokines-related pathological mechanisms such as dysregulation in oligodendrocytes maintenance, microglial toxicity, and alter myelination [59, 60].

Previous reports linked Alzheimer's disease and polymorphisms in both TLR4 and CD14 genetic codes [61, 62]. Multiple forms of aggregated α-synuclein, a pathological feature of neurodegenerative diseases, can trigger and activate different TLRs. This indicates that TLRs contribute to the pathology of psychiatric and neurodegenerative diseases. Behaviorally they are implicated in regulating impulsivity [63]. A previous study linked TLR4 and the Gamma-aminobutyric acid (GABA), the principal inhibitory neurotransmitter in the brain, and the GABAergic inhibitory neurons release it. It was reported that the alpha-2 GABAergic receptor activation of the TLR4 is essential in mediating impulsivity. The co-immunoprecipitation of the alpha-2 GABAergic and TLR4 in the ventral tegmental area leads to Cyclic adenosine monophosphate (cAMP) activation. The cAMP translocation activates the cAMP-response element-binding protein (CREB), subsequently stimulating the tyrosine hydroxylase and the corticotropin-releasing factor. Interestingly, the stereotaxic infusion of alpha-2 GABAergic and TLR4 siRNA in herpes simplex virus vector in the ventral tegmental area prevented alcohol and nicotine seeking. Indicating that TLR4 is involved mechanistically in regulating drug abuse mechanisms [64]. GABAergic synapses are modulated by TLR4 signaling. Stimulation of TLR4 by the administration of Lipopolysaccharide (LPS) alters both pre and postsynaptic function of the GABAergic system. The study indicated that both the synthesis and the reuptake of GABA are altered. Electrophysiological recordings have shown that Lipopolysaccharide's administration reduces the miniature inhibitory postsynaptic currents in acute slices, and this inhibition is mediated through the microglia [56]. Another study linked the GABAergic system to TLR in their report pharmacological activation of the GABAB receptor (baclofen) reduced TLR3- and TLR4 mediated inflammation in primary glial cell lines. Similar findings were observed in the expression of TLR3 in blood mononuclear cells isolated from multiple sclerosis patients [65]. Indicating the existence of complex interaction between microglia, TLR4, and GABAergic system.

Besides, activation of TLR4 could interfere with addiction and drug abuse through another mechanism. In another report, it was indicated that pharmacological application of opiate antagonists (naloxone and naltrexone) prevented the TLR4 signaling achieved in LPS treated rodents. Both naloxone and naltrexone have been shown to non stereoselectively inhibit TLR4 [66].

On the other hand, studies have linked TLR signaling and neurodevelopmental disorders such as Autism spectrum disorders [67, 68]. An impairment identifies these disorders in sociability, communication, and characteristics of repetitive behaviors [69]. Accumulated evidence has linked Autism to neuroinflammation. The peripheral level of different TLRs, including TLR2–5 and TLR9, was elevated significantly in autistic patients in clinical settings [70]. In a previous report, flow-cytometric analysis of TLR4/TLR5 and neuregulin 1 - ErbB in the monocytes of schizophrenic and healthy subjects revealed that both TLR4 and TLR5 were elevated where the level of ErbB is reduced significantly in drug-naïve schizophrenic patients compared to healthy controls [67]. Neuregulin 1 – ErbB signaling is crucial in modulating brain development [71]. For example, it is involved in axonal growth [72] and maintenance [73], the expression of acetylcholine receptors [74], electrophysiological firing [75], and synaptic wiring [76]. Cytokine-related mechanisms are unified features of schizophrenia and an emerging hypothesis for the pathology of schizophrenia [77].

The link between TLRs and depression has been identified in both preclinical [78] clinical [79], and postmortem studies [80]. It was further reported that both protein, and mRNA level of TLR2–4, TLR6 and TLR10 was significantly reduced in the prefrontal brain region of depressed suicide subjects compared to the controls [52].

Adult neurogenesis is a physiological process essential for cognitive capacity, learning and memory, synaptic plasticity, modulating mood, and other processes [81, 82]. Dysregulation in adult neurogenesis is linked to schizophrenia [83], Alzheimer's [84], Parkinson's [85], and autism [86]. In TLR2-mutant mice, adult hippocampal neurogenesis was altered. Proliferative cells that are BrdU/doublecortin positive cells were significantly reduced in TLR2-mutant mice. *In Vitro* studies showed that activation of TLR2 enhances the differentiation of neural stem/progenitor cells [87].

4. Pharmacological modulation of TLRs

The pharmacological targeting of TLR has emerged as an appealing strategy for many reasons. First, they are an essential part of the innate immune system responsible for the initiation of the immune response [88]. Also, studies indicated that TLRs modulate the homeostasis [89], neuronal morphogenesis [90, 91], and neurogenesis [87]. Additionally, it was reported that TLRs are implicated in the pathology of multiple brain disorders such as depression [92], Alzheimer [93], Parkinson [94], and ischemia [95]. Molecularly, it is involved in activating one of the key neuronal signaling pathways [96].

Electrophysiological studies have shown that the administration of immunostimulant results in activation of TLR3 alters the expression of AMPAR, decrease the spontaneous firing, and reduce both the frequency and amplitude of mEPSCs [97]. In line with this, the administration of LPS affect the hippocampal neuronal mEPSC both the frequency and amplitude in hippocampal neurons via modulation of TLR4 [98]. Tlr7 knockout mice showed altered hippocampal LTP, an activity-dependent neurophysiological feature, suggesting defects in memory-related functions [99]. Also, Tlr4 mutant mice exhibited an impairment of long-term depression (LTD) in the nucleus accumbens, another activity-dependent neurophysiological feature, suggesting potential alterations in the reward circuitry [100].

Behaviorally, preclinical studies have shown that TLRs' pharmacological modulation is linked to significant phenotypic features of neurological and psychiatric disorders [90]. In a maternal immune activation (MIA) animal model, a valid model for neurodevelopmental psychiatric disorders such as autism and schizophrenia [101], also linked to increased risks for neurodegenerative disorders [102], it was found that the offspring exhibited schizophrenic-like behaviors via modulation of TLR [103], Clinical and preclinical studies have shown that altered TLR pathway is associated with schizophrenic and autism-related behaviors [90, 101, 103–105].

Mice lacking the TLR3 gene exhibited impairment in amygdala-related behaviors and elevated anxiety while performing cued fear-conditioning and elevated plus maze tests [106]. Anatomically, the amygdala is encompassed by a group of subnuclei, more than ten regions [107]. At circuitry level, this brain region receives input from sensory cortical and thalamic areas, which is responsible for the conditioned (CS) and unconditioned stimulus, prefrontal cortex, and hippocampus that mediate the extinction of fear responses and bed nucleus of the stria terminalis (BNST) that coordinate the stress-related responses. Its output is projected to the brainstem, hypothalamic, and cortical areas responsible for emotional responses [108, 109]. The TLR4 mutant mice exhibited altered higher cognitive tasks such as memory retention, acquisition, and contextual fear-learning [110]. The long-term intraventricular infusion with a TLR9 ligand resulted in memory dysfunction and increased risk of neurodegenerative disorders [111].

Prion diseases are a group of progressive neurodegenerative disorders [112], previously it was reported that TLR9 could be involved in the pathology of the progression of prion diseases. A preclinical study has shown that the administration of a TLR 9 ligand, cytosine phosphate guanosine (CpG-ODN) oligodeoxynucleotides, in mice resulted in a significant increase in the survival rate. Suggesting that the activation of TLRs in neurodegenerative diseases could be attributed to neuroprotective mechanisms that involve eliminating of neurotoxic misfolded proteins, which may prove to be a possible therapeutic strategy to the prion diseases [113]. This immunostimulant has been employed and examined in infectious, allergies ad cancer-related studies [114].

Similarly, genetic therapy targeting TLR2 reduces the accumulation of Amyloid β1–42 in the hippocampus of an animal model of Alzheimer's disease and alters the progression of memory loss [115]. Misfolded α-synuclein is a characteristic feature and a leading cause of neurodegenerative diseases. Employment of immunization has gained a lot of attention as an attractive therapeutic option for neurodegenerative disorders. In a transgenic mice model of Parkinson's, it was found that the immunization with human α-synuclein associated with a marked reduction in the accumulated α-Synuclein and overall reduced neurodegeneration. Indicating that α-Synuclein vaccination could be efficient in reducing neurodegeneration associated with accumulated α-Synuclein [116].

A recent study has reported that treating Parkinson's mice model with a natural compound, Juglanin, lead to enhanced memory function, reduced amyloid-beta accumulation, reversed α-synuclein accumulation and overall anti-inflammatory, and antioxidant effects through the modulation of TLR4/nuclear factor (NF)-κB pathway in the hippocampus [117]. In a clinical setting, treatment with vinpocetine, an alkaloid derivative and a phosphodiesterase type 1 inhibitor, compared to traditional treatment with levodopa, resulted in a significant reduction of TLR 2,4 mRNA level along with reduced the level of serum inflammatory mediators. Interestingly these alterations were associated with a marked elevation while performing the Mini-Mental State Examination score [118]. Although this study did not elucidate the link between TLR2,4 and the enhanced cognitive capacity, it was reported previously that in a dementia model, vinpocetine modulates long-term potentiation [119], Additionally, vinpocetine was found learning and memory while performing Morris maze tasks in fetal alcohol spectrum disorders mice model [120]. Although this study did not elucidate the link between TLR2,4 and the enhanced cognitive capacity, it was reported previously that in a dementia model, vinpocetine modulates long-term potentiation [119]. Additionally, vinpocetine was found learning and memory while performing Morris maze tasks in fetal alcohol spectrum disorders mice model [120]. Interestingly, previously it was found that the inhibition of Cyclic Nucleotide Phosphodiesterase is associated with an alteration of TLRs signaling, apoptotic pathway, and in chronic lymphocytic leukemia cells [121].

Transgenic animal studies have demonstrated that genetic manipulation of TLRs is associated with increased aggravated of Aβ [122]. Treatment with an anti-TLR2 antibody has found to be an effective strategy in providing significant protection preclinically against sepsis-associated death [123], stroke [124], Alzheimer's [123], and its safety, tolerability, along with pharmacokinetic profiling have been conducted clinically in healthy subjects [125]. A 7-month administration of anti-TLR2 antibody to an Alzheimer mice model, APP/PS1 Mice, resulted in an overall reduction in the activation of both microglial and astroglia. This reduction was detected by quantifying immunoreactive MHCII, CD68 (microglial markers), and GFAP (astroglia marker) positive cells. Along with a marked reduction in Ab plaque burden in the hippocampal brain region. Behaviorally, the chronic treatment with TLR2 antibody has improved their performance in water maze test, and the latency was reduced significantly, and the time spent in the platform zone [126].

Studies have linked vitamin D deficiency and increased risk of neurodegenerative diseases [127, 128]. In MPTP (1-methyl-4-phenyl-1,2,3,6-tetrahydropyridine)-Parkinson's induced mouse model treatment with vitamin D has shown notable attenuated nigrostriatal neurodegeneration. Additionally, it increased the tyrosine hydrolase neuronal cells, altered the expression of Iba1 positive cells (microglial activation marker), and TLR-4 [129]. In another study, the same model has employed and treated with Rosmarinus acid, a phenolic compound with anti-oxidant, anti-apoptotic, and anti-inflammatory effects [130]. In a dose-dependent manner, Rosmarinus acid treatment led to a significant improvement of motor dysfunction, elevated the number of tyrosine hydroxylase-positive cells, and downregulated TLR4 [131].

In a rat model of subarachnoid hemorrhage, pharmacological application of a natural flavonoid (Fisetin) minimizes the brain edema, improved modulate neurological scores, and modulate apoptosis, mainly through the regulation of TLR 4/NF-κB signaling [132]. Taken together, the TLR pathway is an attractive candidate for the development of future neurodegenerative therapies.

5. Conclusion

TLRs contribute to modulate physiological and pathological processes. Besides, immunomodulation of TLRs seems to be a promising strategy. More studies are needed to decipher the molecular, cellular, and functional mechanisms involved in modulating proper brain function. Understanding such mechanisms would significantly clarify the complex nature of brain disorders. On broader aspects, mechanistic studies would facilitate finding the best therapeutic intervention for neurodegenerative and psychiatric diseases.

Acknowledgements

The authors extend their appreciation to the Deputyship for Research and Innovation of the Ministry of Education in Saudi Arabia for funding this research work through the project number IFKSURP- 332.

The authors extend their appreciation to the Mentoring Track program.

Conflict of interest

The authors declare no conflict of interest.

Author details

Tahani K. Alshammari[1*], Nouf M. Alrasheed[1], Lina Alhushan[2], Reema Alhoutah[2], Anfal F. Bin Dayel[1], Asma S. Alonazi[1] and Musaad A. Alshammari[1]

1 Department of Pharmacology and Toxicology, College of Pharmacy, King Saud University, Riyadh, Saudi Arabia

2 College of Pharmacy, King Saud University, Riyadh, Saudi Arabia

*Address all correspondence to: talshammary@ksu.edu.sa

References

[1] Amor, S., et al., Inflammation in neurodegenerative diseases. Immunology, 2010.129(2): p. 154-169.

[2] Rhie, S.J., E.-Y. Jung, and I. Shim, The role of neuroinflammation on pathogenesis of affective disorders. Journal of exercise rehabilitation, 2020.16(1): p. 2-9.

[3] Kempuraj, D., et al., Neuroinflammation Induces Neurodegeneration. Journal of neurology, neurosurgery and spine, 2016. 1(1): p. 1003.

[4] Newcombe, E.A., et al., Inflammation: The link between comorbidities, genetics, and Alzheimer's disease. Journal of Neuroinflammation, 2018. 15(1): p. 276.

[5] Duric, V., et al., Comorbidity factors and brain mechanisms linking chronic stress and systemic illness. Neural Plasticity, 2016. 2016: p. 5460732.

[6] Dregan, A., et al., Common mental disorders within chronic inflammatory disorders: A primary care database prospective investigation. Annals of the Rheumatic Diseases, 2019. 78(5): p. 688.

[7] Finnell, J.E. and S.K. Wood, Neuroinflammation at the interface of depression and cardiovascular disease: Evidence from rodent models of social stress. Neurobiology of Stress, 2016. 4: p. 1-14.

[8] Tufekci, K.U., S. Genc, and K. Genc, The endotoxin-induced Neuroinflammation model of Parkinson's disease. Parkinson's 2019 Disease, 2011. 2011: p. 487450.

[9] Adzic, M., et al., Therapeutic strategies for treatment of inflammation-related depression. Current neuropharmacology, 2018. 16(2): p. 176-209.

[10] Glass, C.K., et al., Mechanisms underlying inflammation in neurodegeneration. Cell, 2010. 140(6): p. 918-934.

[11] Paul, B.D., S.H. Snyder, and V.A. Bohr, Signaling by cGAS-STING in neurodegeneration, Neuroinflammation, and aging. Trends Neurosci, 2021. 44(2): p. 83-96.

[12] Butchi, N.B., et al., TLR7 and TLR9 trigger distinct neuroinflammatory responses in the CNS. The American journal of pathology, 2011. 179(2): p. 783-794.

[13] Kim, D.R., T.L. Bale, and C.N. Epperson, Prenatal programming of mental illness: Current understanding of relationship and mechanisms. Current psychiatry reports, 2015. 17(2): p. 5-5.

[14] Brown, A.S. and E.J. Derkits, Prenatal infection and schizophrenia: A review of epidemiologic and translational studies. Am J Psychiatry, 2010. 167(3): p. 261-280.

[15] Younga H. Lee, et al., Maternal bacterial infection during pregnancy and offspring risk of psychotic disorders: Variation by severity of infection and offspring sex. American Journal of Psychiatry, 2020. 177(1): p. 66-75.

[16] McDermott, S., et al., Urinary tract infections during pregnancy and mental retardation and developmental delay. Obstet Gynecol, 2000. 96(1): p. 113-119.

[17] Babulas, V., et al., Prenatal exposure to maternal genital and reproductive infections and adult schizophrenia. American Journal of Psychiatry, 2006. 163(5): p. 927-929.

[18] Verlaet, A.A.J., et al., Nutrition, immunological mechanisms and dietary

immunomodulation in ADHD. European Child & Adolescent Psychiatry, 2014. 23(7): p. 519-529.

[19] Anand, D., et al., Attention-deficit/ hyperactivity disorder and inflammation: What does current knowledge tell us? A systematic review. Frontiers in psychiatry, 2017. 8: p. 228-228.

[20] Hung, Y.-F., et al., Endosomal TLR3, TLR7, and TLR8 control neuronal morphology through different transcriptional programs. Journal of Cell Biology, 2018. 217(8): p. 2727-2742.

[21] Cavaillon, J.M., Exotoxins and endotoxins: Inducers of inflammatory cytokines. Toxicon, 2018. 149: p. 45-53.

[22] Fullerton, J.N., et al., Intravenous endotoxin challenge in healthy humans: An experimental platform to investigate and modulate systemic inflammation. Journal of visualized experiments : JoVE, 2016(111): p. 53913.

[23] Seemann, S., F. Zohles, and A. Lupp, Comprehensive comparison of three different animal models for systemic inflammation. Journal of Biomedical Science, 2017. 24(1): p. 60.

[24] Zakaria, R., et al., Lipopolysaccharide-induced memory impairment in rats: A model of Alzheimer's disease. Physiol Res, 2017. 66(4): p. 553-565.

[25] Liu, M. and G. Bing, Lipopolysaccharide Animal Models for Parkinson's Disease. Parkinson's Disease, 2011. 2011: p. 327089.

[26] Cordeiro, R.C., et al., Leptin Prevents Lipopolysaccharide-Induced Depressive-Like Behaviors in Mice: Involvement of Dopamine Receptors. Frontiers in Psychiatry, 2019. 10(125).

[27] Lee, B., et al., Protective effects of quercetin on anxiety-like symptoms and Neuroinflammation induced by lipopolysaccharide in rats. Evidence-Based Complementary and Alternative Medicine, 2020. 2020: p. 4892415.

[28] Brown, G.C., The endotoxin hypothesis of neurodegeneration. Journal of neuroinflammation, 2019. 16(1): p. 180-180.

[29] Sly, L.M., et al., Endogenous brain cytokine mRNA and inflammatory responses to lipopolysaccharide are elevated in the Tg2576 transgenic mouse model of Alzheimer's disease. Brain Res Bull, 2001. 56(6): p. 581-588.

[30] Kitazawa, M., et al., Lipopolysaccharide-induced inflammation exacerbates tau pathology by a cyclin-dependent kinase 5-mediated pathway in a transgenic model of Alzheimer's disease. J Neurosci, 2005. 25(39): p. 8843-8853.

[31] Lalioti, V., D. Pulido, and I.V. Sandoval, Cdk5, the multifunctional surveyor. Cell Cycle, 2010. 9(2): p. 284-311.

[32] Lopes, J.P. and P. Agostinho, Cdk5: Multitasking between physiological and pathological conditions. Prog Neurobiol, 2011. 94(1): p. 49-63.

[33] Cheung, Z.H., A.K. Fu, and N.Y. Ip, Synaptic roles of Cdk5: Implications in higher cognitive functions and neurodegenerative diseases. Neuron, 2006. 50(1): p. 13-18.

[34] Cheung, Z.H. and N.Y. Ip, Cdk5: Mediator of neuronal death and survival. Neurosci Lett, 2004. 361(1-3): p. 47-51.

[35] Wilkaniec, A., et al., Inhibition of cyclin-dependent kinase 5 affects early neuroinflammatory signalling in murine model of amyloid beta toxicity. Journal of Neuroinflammation, 2018. 15(1): p. 1.

[36] Jaeger, L.B., et al., Lipopolysaccharide alters the blood-brain barrier transport of amyloid beta protein: A mechanism for inflammation in the progression of Alzheimer's disease. Brain Behav Immun, 2009. 23(4): p. 507-517.

[37] Qin, L., et al., NADPH oxidase and aging drive microglial activation, oxidative stress, and dopaminergic neurodegeneration following systemic LPS administration. Glia, 2013. 61(6): p. 855-868.

[38] Mangano, E.N. and S. Hayley, Inflammatory priming of the substantia nigra influences the impact of later paraquat exposure: Neuroimmune sensitization of neurodegeneration. Neurobiology of Aging, 2009. 30(9): p. 1361-1378.

[39] Kiecolt-Glaser, J.K., et al., Marital distress, depression, and a leaky gut: Translocation of bacterial endotoxin as a pathway to inflammation. Psychoneuroendocrinology, 2018. 98: p. 52-60.

[40] van den Boogaard, M., et al., Endotoxemia-induced inflammation and the effect on the human brain. Crit Care, 2010. 14(3): p. R81.

[41] Kullmann, J.S., et al., Neural response to emotional stimuli during experimental human endotoxemia. Hum Brain Mapp, 2013. 34(9): p. 2217-2227.

[42] Sayk, F., et al., Endotoxemia causes central downregulation of sympathetic vasomotor tone in healthy humans. Am J Physiol Regul Integr Comp Physiol, 2008. 295(3): p. R891-R898.

[43] Moieni, M., et al., Inflammation impairs social cognitive processing: A randomized controlled trial of endotoxin. Brain Behav Immun, 2015. 48: p. 132-138.

[44] Schmahl, C., et al., Mechanisms of disturbed emotion processing and social interaction in borderline personality disorder: State of knowledge and research agenda of the German clinical research unit. Borderline personality disorder and emotion dysregulation, 2014. 1: p. 12-12.

[45] Trivedi, J.K., Cognitive deficits in psychiatric disorders: Current status. Indian journal of psychiatry, 2006. 48(1): p. 10-20.

[46] Etkin, A., A. Gyurak, and R. O'Hara, A neurobiological approach to the cognitive deficits of psychiatric disorders. Dialogues in clinical neuroscience, 2013. 15(4): p. 419-429.

[47] Fernandes, J.M., et al., Social cognition in schizophrenia and autism Spectrum disorders: A systematic review and meta-analysis of direct comparisons. Frontiers in psychiatry, 2018. 9: p. 504-504.

[48] Irwin, M.R., et al., Moderators for depressed mood and systemic and transcriptional inflammatory responses: A randomized controlled trial of endotoxin. Neuropsychopharmacology, 2019. 44(3): p. 635-641.

[49] Hannestad, J., et al., Citalopram reduces endotoxin-induced fatigue. Brain Behav Immun, 2011. 25(2): p. 256-259.

[50] Zhang, R., et al., Circulating endotoxin and systemic immune activation in sporadic amyotrophic lateral sclerosis (sALS). J Neuroimmunol, 2009. 206(1-2): p. 121-124.

[51] Kouli, A., C.B. Horne, and C.H. Williams-Gray, Toll-like receptors and their therapeutic potential in Parkinson's disease and α-synucleinopathies. Brain Behav Immun, 2019. 81: p. 41-51.

[52] Pandey, G.N., et al., Innate immunity in the postmortem brain of depressed and suicide subjects: Role of toll-like receptors. Brain Behav Immun, 2019. 75: p. 101-111.

[53] Martín-Hernández, D., et al., Intracellular inflammatory and antioxidant pathways in postmortem frontal cortex of subjects with major depression: Effect of antidepressants. Journal of Neuroinflammation, 2018. 15(1): p. 251.

[54] Zhou, Z., et al., Toll-like receptor-mediated immune responses in intestinal macrophages; implications for mucosal immunity and autoimmune diseases. Clinical immunology (Orlando, Fla.), 2016. 173: p. 81-86.

[55] Burgueño, J.F., et al., TLR2 and TLR9 modulate enteric nervous system inflammatory responses to lipopolysaccharide. Journal of Neuroinflammation, 2016. 13(1): p. 187.

[56] Yan, X., E. Jiang, and H.-R. Weng, Activation of toll like receptor 4 attenuates GABA synthesis and postsynaptic GABA receptor activities in the spinal dorsal horn via releasing interleukin-1 beta. Journal of neuroinflammation, 2015. 12: p. 222-222.

[57] Crowley, T., et al., Modulation of TLR3/TLR4 inflammatory signaling by the GABAB receptor agonist baclofen in glia and immune cells: relevance to therapeutic effects in multiple sclerosis. Frontiers in Cellular Neuroscience, 2015. 9(284).

[58] Kim, J.K., et al., GABAergic signaling linked to autophagy enhances host protection against intracellular bacterial infections. Nature Communications, 2018. 9(1): p. 4184.

[59] Hanke, M.L. and T. Kielian, Toll-like receptors in health and disease in the brain: mechanisms and therapeutic potential. Clinical science (London, England: 1979), 2011. 121(9): p. 367-387.

[60] Lacagnina, M.J., L.R. Watkins, and P.M. Grace, Toll-like receptors and their role in persistent pain. Pharmacology & therapeutics, 2018. 184: p. 145-158.

[61] Balistreri, C.R., et al., Association between the polymorphisms of TLR4 and CD14 genes and Alzheimer's disease. Curr Pharm Des, 2008. 14(26): p. 2672-2677.

[62] Rodríguez-Fandiño, O., J. Hernández-Ruiz, and M. Schmulson, From cytokines to toll-like receptors and beyond - current knowledge and future research needs in irritable bowel syndrome. Journal of neurogastroenterology and motility, 2010. 16(4): p. 363-373.

[63] Aurelian, L., et al., TLR4 signaling in VTA dopaminergic neurons regulates impulsivity through tyrosine hydroxylase modulation. Transl Psychiatry, 2016. 6(5): p. e815.

[64] Balan, I., et al., The GABA(a) receptor α2 subunit activates a neuronal TLR4 signal in the ventral tegmental area that regulates alcohol and nicotine abuse. Brain sciences, 2018. 8(4): p. 72.

[65] Crowley, T., et al., Modulation of TLR3/TLR4 inflammatory signaling by the GABAB receptor agonist baclofen in glia and immune cells: Relevance to therapeutic effects in multiple sclerosis. Frontiers in cellular neuroscience, 2015. 9: p. 284-284.

[66] Skolnick, P., et al., Translational potential of naloxone and naltrexone as TLR4 antagonists. Trends Pharmacol Sci, 2014. 35(9): p. 431-432.

[67] Kéri, S., C. Szabó, and O. Kelemen, Uniting the neurodevelopmental and immunological hypotheses: Neuregulin 1 receptor ErbB and toll-like receptor

activation in first-episode schizophrenia. Scientific Reports, 2017. 7(1): p. 4147.

[68] Ratnayake, U., et al., Cytokines and the neurodevelopmental basis of mental illness. Frontiers in Neuroscience, 2013. 7(180).

[69] Mahmood, H.M., et al., The role of nicotinic receptors in the attenuation of autism-related behaviors in a murine BTBR T + tf/J autistic model. Autism Res, 2020. 13(8): p. 1311-1334.

[70] Enstrom, A.M., et al., Differential monocyte responses to TLR ligands in children with autism spectrum disorders. Brain Behav Immun, 2010. 24(1): p. 64-71.

[71] Corfas, G., K. Roy, and J.D. Buxbaum, Neuregulin 1-erbB signaling and the molecular/cellular basis of schizophrenia. Nat Neurosci, 2004. 7(6): p. 575-580.

[72] Heermann, S., et al., Neuregulin 1 type III/ErbB signaling is crucial for Schwann cell colonization of sympathetic axons. PLOS ONE, 2011. 6(12): p. e28692.

[73] Rao, S.N.R. and D.D. Pearse, Regulating axonal responses to injury: The intersection between signaling pathways involved in axon myelination and the inhibition of axon regeneration. Frontiers in molecular neuroscience, 2016. 9: p. 33-33.

[74] Hancock, M.L., et al., Presynaptic type III neuregulin1-ErbB signaling targets {alpha}7 nicotinic acetylcholine receptors to axons. The Journal of cell biology, 2008. 181(3): p. 511-521.

[75] Chen, Y.-J., et al., ErbB4 in parvalbumin-positive interneurons is critical for neuregulin 1 regulation of long-term potentiation. Proceedings of the National Academy of Sciences, 2010. 107(50): p. 21818.

[76] Mei, L. and W.C. Xiong, Neuregulin 1 in neural development, synaptic plasticity and schizophrenia. Nat Rev Neurosci, 2008. 9(6): p. 437-452.

[77] Girgis, R.R., S.S. Kumar, and A.S. Brown, The cytokine model of schizophrenia: Emerging therapeutic strategies. Biological Psychiatry, 2014. 75(4): p. 292-299.

[78] Gárate, I., et al., Origin and consequences of brain toll-like receptor 4 pathway stimulation in an experimental model of depression. Journal of Neuroinflammation, 2011. 8(1): p. 151.

[79] Hung, Y.-Y., et al., Association between toll-likc receptors expression and major depressive disorder. Psychiatry Research, 2014. 220(1): p. 283-286.

[80] Pandey, G.N., et al., Toll-like receptors in the depressed and suicide brain. J Psychiatr Res, 2014. 53: p. 62-68.

[81] Toda, T., et al., The role of adult hippocampal neurogenesis in brain health and disease. Molecular psychiatry, 2019. 24(1): p. 67-87.

[82] Zhao, C., W. Deng, and F.H. Gage, Mechanisms and functional implications of adult neurogenesis. Cell, 2008. 132(4): p. 645-660.

[83] Hong, S., et al., Defective neurogenesis and schizophrenia-like behavior in PARP-1-deficient mice. Cell Death & Disease, 2019. 10(12): p. 943.

[84] Rodríguez, J.J. and A. Verkhratsky, Neurogenesis in Alzheimer's disease. J Anat, 2011. 219(1): p. 78-89.

[85] Marxreiter, F., M. Regensburger, and J. Winkler, Adult neurogenesis in Parkinson's disease. Cell Mol Life Sci, 2013. 70(3): p. 459-473.

[86] Gilbert, J. and H.-Y. Man, Fundamental elements in autism:

From neurogenesis and neurite growth to synaptic plasticity. Frontiers in cellular neuroscience, 2017. 11: p. 359-359.

[87] Rolls, A., et al., Toll-like receptors modulate adult hippocampal neurogenesis. Nat Cell Biol, 2007. 9(9): p. 1081-1088.

[88] Rietdijk, C.D., et al., Neuronal toll-like receptors and neuro-immunity in Parkinson's disease, Alzheimer's disease and stroke. Neuroimmunology and Neuroinflammation, 2016. 3: p. 27-37.

[89] Kielian, T., Toll-like receptors in central nervous system glial inflammation and homeostasis. Journal of Neuroscience Research, 2006. 83(5): p. 711-730.

[90] Chen, C.Y., et al., Beyond defense: Regulation of neuronal morphogenesis and brain functions via toll-like receptors. J Biomed Sci, 2019. 26(1): p. 90.

[91] Kaul, D., et al., Expression of toll-like receptors in the developing brain. PLoS One, 2012. 7(5): p. e37767.

[92] Alshammari, T.K., et al., Assessing the role of toll-like receptor in isolated, standard and enriched housing conditions. PLoS One, 2019. 14(10): p. e0222818.

[93] Gambuzza, M.E., et al., Toll-like receptors in Alzheimer's disease: A therapeutic perspective. CNS Neurol Disord Drug Targets, 2014. 13(9): p. 1542-1558.

[94] Beraud, D. and K.A. Maguire-Zeiss, Misfolded alpha-synuclein and toll-like receptors: Therapeutic targets for Parkinson's disease. Parkinsonism Relat Disord, 2012. 18 Suppl 1: p. S17-S20.

[95] Tang, S.C., et al., Pivotal role for neuronal toll-like receptors in ischemic brain injury and functional deficits. Proc Natl Acad Sci U S A, 2007. 104(34): p. 13798-13803.

[96] Sai-Yu Hou, T.-L.H.C.-C.L.; Ming-Kung Wu;Yi-Yung Hung, Effects of Selective Serotonin Reuptake Inhibitors and Serotonin-Norepinephrine Reuptake Inhibitors on Toll-Like-Receptors Expression Profiles. Neuropsychiatry, 2018. 8(1): p. 243-248.

[97] Ritchie, L., et al., Toll-like receptor 3 activation impairs excitability and synaptic activity via TRIF signalling in immature rat and human neurons. Neuropharmacology, 2018. 135: p. 1-10.

[98] Shen, Y., et al., Postnatal activation of TLR4 in astrocytes promotes excitatory synaptogenesis in hippocampal neurons. J Cell Biol, 2016. 215(5): p. 719-734.

[99] Hung, Y.F., et al., Tlr7 deletion alters expression profiles of genes related to neural function and regulates mouse behaviors and contextual memory. Brain Behav Immun, 2018. 72: p. 101-113.

[100] Kashima, D.T. and B.A. Grueter, Toll-like receptor 4 deficiency alters nucleus accumbens synaptic physiology and drug reward behavior. Proc Natl Acad Sci U S A, 2017. 114(33): p. 8865-8870.

[101] Conway, F. and A.S. Brown, Maternal immune activation and related factors in the risk of offspring psychiatric disorders. Front Psychiatry, 2019. 10: p. 430.

[102] Knuesel, I., et al., Maternal immune activation and abnormal brain development across CNS disorders. Nat Rev Neurol, 2014. 10(11): p. 643-660.

[103] Reisinger, S., et al., The poly(I:C)-induced maternal immune activation model in preclinical neuropsychiatric drug discovery. Pharmacol Ther, 2015. 149: p. 213-226.

[104] Missig, G., et al., Sex-dependent neurobiological features of prenatal immune activation via TLR7. Mol Psychiatry, 2019.

[105] Kéri, S., C. Szabó, and O. Kelemen, Antipsychotics influence toll-like receptor (TLR) expression and its relationship with cognitive functions in schizophrenia. Brain Behav Immun, 2017. 62: p. 256-264.

[106] Okun, E., et al., Toll-like receptor 3 inhibits memory retention and constrains adult hippocampal neurogenesis. Proc Natl Acad Sci U S A, 2010. 107(35): p. 15625-15630.

[107] Davis, M., The role of the amygdala in conditioned fear, in The amygdala: Neurobiological aspects of emotion, memory, and mental dysfunction. 1992, Wiley-Liss: New York, NY, USA. p. 255-306.

[108] Ressler, K.J., Amygdala activity, fear, and anxiety: Modulation by stress. Biol Psychiatry, 2010. 67(12): p. 1117-1119.

[109] Janak, P.H. and K.M. Tye, From circuits to behaviour in the amygdala. Nature, 2015. 517(7534): p. 284-292.

[110] Okun, E., et al., Evidence for a developmental role for TLR4 in learning and memory. PLoS One, 2012. 7(10): p. e47522.

[111] Tauber, S.C., et al., Stimulation of toll-like receptor 9 by chronic intraventricular unmethylated cytosine-guanine DNA infusion causes neuroinflammation and impaired spatial memory. J Neuropathol Exp Neurol, 2009. 68(10): p. 1116-1124.

[112] Prusiner, S.B., Neurodegenerative diseases and prions. New England Journal of Medicine, 2001. 344(20): p. 1516-1526.

[113] Sethi, S., et al., Postexposure prophylaxis against prion disease with a stimulator of innate immunity. Lancet, 2002. 360(9328): p. 229-230.

[114] Lai, C.Y., et al., Immunostimulatory activities of CpG-Oligodeoxynucleotides in Teleosts: Toll-like receptors 9 and 21. Front Immunol, 2019. 10: p. 179.

[115] Richard, K.L., et al., Toll-like receptor 2 acts as a natural innate immune receptor to clear amyloid β_{1-42} and delay the cognitive decline in a mouse model of Alzheimer's disease. The Journal of Neuroscience, 2008. 28(22): p. 5784-5793.

[116] Masliah, E., et al., Effects of alpha-synuclein immunization in a mouse model of Parkinson's disease. Neuron, 2005. 46(6): p. 857-868.

[117] Zhang, F.X. and R.S. Xu, Juglanin ameliorates LPS-induced neuroinflammation in animal models of Parkinson's disease and cell culture via inactivating TLR4/NF-kappaB pathway. Biomed Pharmacother, 2018. 97: p. 1011-1019.

[118] Ping, Z., et al., Vinpocetine regulates levels of circulating TLRs in Parkinson's disease patients. Neurol Sci, 2019. 40(1): p. 113-120.

[119] Molnar, P., L. Gaal, and C. Horvath, The impairment of long-term potentiation in rats with medial septal lesion and its restoration by cognition enhancers. Neurobiology (Bp), 1994. 2(3): p. 255-266.

[120] Filgueiras, C.C., T.E. Krahe, and A.E. Medina, Phosphodiesterase type 1 inhibition improves learning in rats exposed to alcohol during the third trimester equivalent of human gestation. Neurosci Lett, 2010. 473(3): p. 202-207.

[121] Tan, Y., et al., Inhibition of type 4 cyclic nucleotide phosphodiesterase blocks intracellular TLR signaling in chronic lymphocytic leukemia and

normal hematopoietic cells. J Immunol, 2015. 194(1): p. 101-112.

[122] Tahara, K., et al., Role of toll-like receptor signalling in Abeta uptake and clearance. Brain, 2006. 129(Pt 11): p. 3006-3019.

[123] Lima, C.X., et al., Therapeutic effects of treatment with anti-TLR2 and anti-TLR4 monoclonal antibodies in Polymicrobial sepsis. PLoS One, 2015. 10(7): p. e0132336.

[124] Brea, D., et al., Toll-like receptors 2 and 4 in ischemic stroke: Outcome and therapeutic values. J Cereb Blood Flow Metab, 2011. 31(6): p. 1424-1431.

[125] Reilly, M., et al., Randomized, double-blind, placebo-controlled, dose-escalating phase I, healthy subjects study of intravenous OPN-305, a humanized anti-TLR2 antibody. Clin Pharmacol Ther, 2013. 94(5): p. 593-600.

[126] McDonald, C.L., et al., Inhibiting TLR2 activation attenuates amyloid accumulation and glial activation in a mouse model of Alzheimer's disease. Brain Behav Immun, 2016. 58: p. 191-200.

[127] Chai, B., et al., Vitamin D deficiency as a risk factor for dementia and Alzheimer's disease: An updated meta-analysis. BMC Neurology, 2019. 19(1): p. 284.

[128] Banerjee, A., et al., Vitamin D and Alzheimer's Disease: Neurocognition to Therapeutics. International Journal of Alzheimer's Disease, 2015. 2015: p. 192747.

[129] Calvello, R., et al., Vitamin D treatment attenuates Neuroinflammation and dopaminergic neurodegeneration in an animal model of Parkinson's disease, shifting M1 to M2 microglia responses. J Neuroimmune Pharmacol, 2017. 12(2): p. 327-339.

[130] Luo, C., et al., A review of the anti-inflammatory effects of Rosmarinic acid on inflammatory diseases. Front Pharmacol, 2020. 11: p. 153.

[131] Lv, R., et al., Rosmarinic acid attenuates inflammatory responses through inhibiting HMGB1/TLR4/NF-kappaB signaling pathway in a mouse model of Parkinson's disease. Life Sci, 2019. 223: p. 158-165.

[132] Zhou, C.H., et al., Fisetin alleviates early brain injury following experimental subarachnoid hemorrhage in rats possibly by suppressing TLR 4/NF-kappaB signaling pathway. Brain Res, 2015. 1629: p. 250-259.